Bedded Bliss

Bedded Bliss

A COUPLE'S GUIDE TO LUST EVER AFTER

KRISTINA WRIGHT

FOREWORD BY
MARK A. MICHAELS AND PATRICIA JOHNSON

PRESS

Published in the United States by Cleis Press, Inc., 2246 Sixth Street, Berkeley, California 94710.

Printed in the United States.
Cover design: Scott Idleman/Blink
Cover photograph: Melissa Scheetz/Getty Images
Text design: Frank Wiedemann

First Edition.
10 9 8 7 6 5 4 3 2 1

Trade paper ISBN: 978-1-57344-964-9
E-book ISBN: 978-1-57344-979-3

Library of Congress Cataloging-in-Publication Data

Bedded bliss : a couple's guide to lust ever after / [edited by] Kristina Wright. -- First edition.
     pages cm
ISBN 978-1-57344-964-9 (alk. paper)
1. Erotic stories, American. I. Wright, Kristina, editor of compilation.

PS648.E7B425 2013
813'.01083538--dc23

                              2013026048

For Jay,
always and forever

CONTENTS

CONTENTS

CONTENTS

FOREWORD

MARK A. MICHAELS AND PATRICIA JOHNSON

edded Bliss is an important and delightful book, one that successfully fuses two genres that are not easily combined: self-help and erotica. Great insights into the nature of long-term love are accompanied by stories that combine sexual heat and emotional intimacy in ways that are often interesting and surprising. The stories and anecdotes are sure to fuel your erotic imagination, even if you are in a newer relationship.

We have been lovers for over fourteen years and will be celebrating our thirteenth wedding anniversary in just a few months. We got together with no intention of becoming a couple, and we didn't even date, at least not in the conventional sense. We met at Mark's first public lecture on Tantra, exchanged emails for a few weeks, and then went out for lunch. Over that first meal, we decided to practice sexual Tantra together, with no expectations that we would fall in love, let alone become life partners. Thus, sex has been central to our partnership from the start. It's also our profession, so most of our days involve discussing, teaching, researching, writing and thinking about sex.

The more we learn, the more we realize how little we know. Perhaps more importantly, even though sex and relationships are so central to our lives, we still have to resist the temptation to fall into ruts, to take each other for granted, to make love less frequently than we could or should. This is bound to happen in any partnership that has endured beyond the often tumultuous and heady state that is sometimes called "new relationship energy." In the early stages, new relationship energy is a powerful driving force, so compelling that there's little need to think about sex, let alone make an effort to have it. Similarly, new relationships typically don't need tending outside the bedroom; the intensity of the emotions alone is usually enough to keep partners focused on each other. *Bedded Bliss* reminds us that there's always room to be more attentive to our partnership and to our sexual life together.

In time, the intensity of being in a new relationship must fade, and the quantity, but not necessarily the quality, of sex is likely to decrease. This evolution is often represented as being tragic—*Romeo and Juliet* can be read as a metaphor for the death of new relationship energy—or if not tragic, as the beginning of a new phase in which boredom is bound to set in. In this domestic phase, boredom is often presented as if it were the best possible outcome. The *"Married with Children"* model is equally common and even more toxic—long-term partnership as a kind of endless, low intensity war. The positive alternatives to these negative representations tend to be generic—"they lived happily ever after"—which implies that good relationships take care of themselves and that what is really a beginning is a culmination. The truth is that relationships require nurturing and attention; we have described ourselves as "a devoted married couple" for many years. Our choice of the word "devoted" is deliberate. It reflects our belief that a partnership is something that merits your full attention—that the person with whom you've chosen to spend your life deserves to be honored and embraced.

This core principle is woven into every anecdote and every story in *Bedded Bliss*. Partners turn toward each other, emotionally and erotically, even during difficult times. They decide again and again to be sexual, even when the "mood" isn't there or when they're feeling stressed. There are bittersweet moments; there are deep insights; there's an appreciation for middle-aged sex that's badly needed in a culture that seems to be ever more youth-oriented. There's an awareness that loving sex can be profoundly healing, as in Kristina Wright's moving,

"The Weight of Things." There's also humor, something that's too often absent from books about sex. Having the capacity to laugh at ourselves both in and out of bed is just as important as treating our partners with love and respect.

There's something for everyone in *Bedded Bliss*, and all options are gently presented as potentially valid. For some this may involve kink or some form of open relationship; for others, exclusivity and what sometimes gets denigrated as "vanilla" sex are completely satisfying. There's no one-size-fits-all approach.

Wright astutely observes that sexually satisfied couples are a kind of invisible population. The same can be said about generally happy couples. This is in part because of the way long-term relationships are portrayed, both in popular culture and in literature. It's also due to the fact that many relationship books are written by therapists whose perspective has been shaped by helping couples in crisis. This therapeutic slant may not be of much value for reasonably happy couples seeking to make things better or those facing minor and relatively transitory issues. For couples like these, and even for some facing more serious problems, the best advice may be to focus on the positive—the things that brought you together in the first place, the love you have for each other, the life you've built—and to be intentional about connecting erotically. *Bedded Bliss* will not only fuel your erotic imagination; it will provide you with practical strategies for remaining within or becoming part of that invisible population, one that is just starting to emerge from the shadows.

MAKING LUST LAST

I look back now and I can't believe I took the leap. We were young and crazy and we hardly knew each other. But he was the one. Still is.
—Kristina Wright, married twenty-three years

We were meant to be together. I knew it before she did.
—James Wright, Kristina's husband

W e met in the airport. The first thing I ever said to the man who would become my husband was, "Please tell me your name is Jay." At the time, I was dating his roommate and Jay was doing him a favor and collecting me from the airport since my then-boyfriend had to work. We had spoken on the phone and I had seen one picture of him—beyond that, I didn't know him at all. He will tell you he saw a picture of me and knew we would end up together. In fact, the story goes that he told his roommate, "I'm going to take her away from you." It didn't quite go down like that, but we did end up together despite my doubts about another long-distance relationship. Jay was more of a romantic than me—at least at the beginning. I caught up fast.

No one thought it would last—except us. And the naysayers no longer have anything to say as we have weathered over two decades of marriage, several military moves, close to a dozen deployments and made a home wherever we were, first with a menagerie of pets and then adding two babies to the mix in our forties. Life is crazy, hectic, chaotic. He is at the tail end of his naval career and contemplating life post-retirement, I have a thriving writing and editing career that I cobble together with part-time childcare and late-night, caffeine-induced writing sessions. The kids are growing like weeds, the house is in constant need of some kind of repair and there is always a holiday or birthday or trip around the corner. In other words: it's just life. Not busier—or better—than yours. We pass in the kitchen and grope each other knowing there's nothing we can do about it for another five hours; we send furtive text messages during nap times, "Are they still asleep? Do we have time?" We do what we have to do to fuel the flames of that raging fire we still feel for each other. And so do you.

We are still going strong, and I think it's a hell of an accomplishment for a couple of love-and-lust-struck twentysomethings who hardly knew each other when they got together. We are lucky—but it's not just luck that got us (and keeps us) here. It's dedication and imagination; it's creative use of our free time (and technology). Most of all, it's love— passionate, ongoing, never-fading love. It's an amazing thing we share, and I never take it for granted. And yet, we are invisible in a culture obsessed with sexual scandals, casual hookups, betrayal, infidelity, divorce and midlife crises. Where are the other couples like us—the couples who fell in love, tumbled headfirst into bed and are still there, tangled amongst the sheets, laughing, living and loving, for better or worse, every single day of their lives? Turns out, there are a lot of couples like us. We are here, we are still in love and lust, and we are happy to share our stories, knowledge and advice with others. Sexy, lusty love is a lifelong pursuit for those of us who know the once-in-a-lifetime flash of lightning of young love doesn't die or fade—it grows stronger and becomes the kind of everyday magic on which to build a life together.

When I first conceptualized the book that would become *Bedded Bliss*, it was with the awareness that there haven't been many (if any) books like it. This is a book filled with real-life experiences, sensual fantasies, practical advice, realistic suggestions, a dash of humor, a lot of sexy erotica, a few poignant memoirs and a combined total of over 235 years of long-term relationship experience. This is a book to remind you that—no matter where you are in your life or your relationship—your passion, your imagination, your *need* is still there and very much alive. It's a book to inspire and encourage—to give you some ideas if you feel as if your well of passion and imagination is running dry. We, these talented, inspiring writers and I, are here to remind you of what you already know (even if you sometimes forget): married sex is a grand, amazing adventure from the first heartfelt "I do" to the distant golden years, and everything in between.

I handpicked the authors for this project—all of them are professional writers, many of them are well known in the erotica and erotic romance genres. These are authors who write about sex for a living, yes, but they are also real people with real lives who know what it's like to share a home, a life and a family with another person. They have experienced it all. Every joy, every frustration, every milestone, *everything* a couple can experience. One or more of the baker's dozen of authors in this book has been where you are *right now* in your marriage.

The short stories and memoirs shared here vary in sensuality from sweetly seductive to wildly erotic. These stories—personal, arousing, inspiring—are an opportunity to share a variety of experiences from authors with as varied backgrounds as the readers who hold the book in their hands. Each story opens with an introduction by the author, a personal vignette from the pages of their own lusty lives to remind you that you are not alone; we are in this pursuit of lifetime passion together. Regardless of where you are currently in your relationship, each story has something to offer you—commiseration and inspiration told from personal experience or clever imagination by writers who understand and appreciate the work that goes into sustaining a lifelong commitment. I got to choose the stories you read here and I wanted very real, attainable scenarios for couples who have as complicated lives as my husband and I do. I wanted to be able to read this book myself and say, "Oh wow, I'm going to try that." (And I'll tell you a secret: that's exactly what happened.) I wanted a book for people like me—with a full life and a busy schedule and a to-do list longer than my arm—who already know that married sex is the *best* sex.

I invite you to share the book with your partner, read the stories together (or out loud to each other) and create some new memories of your own. No matter where you are in your own relationship—if you're years from having kids (or chose to skip that stage entirely) or the newlywed days seem long ago—the stories will offer you a glimpse into the possibilities of your passionate future and remind you of your lusty past—not to mention give you some very sexy scenarios to consider. We've been there, we are there, we are living and loving and lusting and fucking with the person who set us on fire and still stokes our flames. Live that life of bedded bliss you daydreamed about on lazy Sundays on that hand-me-down couch and in late-night whispers before you fell asleep. Never, ever let it go.

I invite you to consider this book not as a self-help book, but as a book of sexy, encouraging cheers. You're already there, sharing your life and bed with the person who rocks your world like no one else. Whatever happens, you're in it together, forever. If you need a little cheer to get you motivated now and again, look here. Choose a fantasy, create your own. You're on the same team and we're on your side, shaking our pom-poms and reminding you that married sex is great and happily ever after exists: you have it. It's right in front of you. Enjoy *every* lusty minute of it.

Yours in bedded bliss,
Kristina Wright

ONE

THE BEGINNING OF LUST—
HOW IT STARTS, WHY IT LASTS

Grow old along with me! The best is yet to be...
—Robert Browning to his wife Elizabeth Barrett
Browning, married fifteen years

*Y*ou knew it was right when you met your partner. Maybe it wasn't love at first sight—maybe it wasn't even love at fiftieth sight—but at some point, you knew this was *the* person you wanted to spend your life with. For me, it wasn't quite love at first sight, but there was definitely an immediate, undeniable connection with the man who would become my husband. If you had told me on January 1 of that first year that I would meet him, fall in love, date long distance and be married before the leaves had fallen from the trees, I would have laughed at you. That kind of magic doesn't exist, does it? Oh, but it does. It's different for everyone, but it's magic when you fall in love. It's magic when you connect on all levels in a way that defies explanation, other than it was simply meant to be. That very real, very profound feeling that brought you together and keeps you together is love. And that hunger for your partner's body, touch, whispered moans and secret fantasies is the lust that drives you into each other's arms to weather any storm, to comfort as only you can, to celebrate again and again the magic that is unique to the two of you.

I remember walking through a museum with my future husband two months after that fateful day we met at the airport. We hadn't seen each other since that first time. He was still my boyfriend's roommate and he had a girlfriend back in Tennessee, but I felt this overwhelming urge to reach out and *touch* him. It wasn't sexual, exactly, but it was something unexpected. I had known there was a physical and intellectual attraction from the first time we met, and that had made it impossible to forget him even though we lived in different states and were both dating other people.

We were just friends, I kept telling myself, and long-distance friends at that. He was smart and funny and chivalrous and cute and he was my *boyfriend's roommate*. Nothing would or could happen. He was safe. He was a nice guy. And yet, I still remember standing next to him at an exhibit in the Smithsonian, the backs of our hands brushing in a way that was equal parts homey comfort and exquisite torture and knowing—just *knowing*—this was the guy. We had only met two months previously and I was getting ready to end my relationship with his roommate for reasons that had nothing to do with this new attraction, but with that simple brush of our hands I knew something wonderful was to be had with this man. Yes, it's corny, I know. Believe me, I was born a cynic and didn't need anyone else to tell me that this kind of thing was fleeting fun, at best. I was convinced it was nothing more than a crush and would fade by the time I got on a plane for home.

Oh, how wrong I was. We stayed up all night talking that night—*just* talking—until the sun rose and our friends woke up and asked if we had slept at all. The sexual tension was so tangible it felt like we shared an exhilarating secret even though we hadn't done anything wrong. A secret between two people who just *got* each other and were meant to be together—eventually. Those months (okay, it was like eight weeks) were the longest months of my life—at least until we got married and he left on a six-month deployment. But shortly after that night, we did end up together and before the year was out, we were married—and I've never looked back.

In whatever form your relationship developed, you had a similar experience of connectedness with your partner. Whether it was a brush of your hands or laughing at the same joke or sharing a meaningful look in a crowded room—there was a point when you looked at each other and you just *knew* this was the person you were going to spend your life loving, between the sheets and otherwise. And whether it took a few weeks or a decade of knowing each other before you committed, once you did you were all in. This is it. This is your life with your partner. It is an amazing feeling, it is a terrifying feeling, it is a roller coaster of ups and downs and promises and memories and history—oh, the history!—of togetherness.

History is a funny thing. It binds us together, giving us shared memories, dirty and otherwise, to keep us connected and in love. But history also has a way of blurring as the years go by, making you forget what it was once like. The fire, the passion, the wildness of that new love. It's still there; it's always there, that hot-bright, magic connection between two people who love each other. In a study that attempts to scientifically prove that love really can last, researchers at the State University of New York at Stony Brook took functional MRI scans of couples married an average of twenty-one years as well as couples in newer relationships. As the participants looked at photos of their partners, the key motivation and reward regions of the brain lit up on their scans, which demonstrated a similar chemistry between the long-married couples and newly coupled pairs.

Love lasts, that's the scientific takeaway, but you don't need a study to tell you what you already know—you feel it all the time. Your focus may shift the longer you're together but it always comes back to center, to the one who keeps you grounded. Life is this constant jumble of commitments and activities and schedules, all of them demanding so much of you and your partner that your connection sometimes runs on autopilot for longer than either of you would like. Then the focus returns, white hot and immediate, and you're right back there, at the beginning, remembering where it all began—and a whole lot more "lights up" than just your brain!

Remember those early days; the way it felt to curl up against each other like two pieces of a puzzle, everything fitting just as it should—like it belonged, because it did. Feeling whole, when you hadn't even realized you felt incomplete. It's still there, that feeling. The way your fingers entwine while you're in the car, the way your face fits in the hollow of his shoulder or the curve of her neck. That instinctive smack on his ass when he bends over to take the roast out of the oven or the tug on her hair, just so, when she's getting ready to come. It's all still there, those feelings so connected to your early days together, it's just become second nature. Instinct. Your partner. *Yours.* Read the stories of lust just taking root, "Take It Off," by Sommer Marsden, and "The Proposal," by Christopher Cole, and remember. This is what it means to be coupled forever, to feel that unconscious pull from across the room and see your love staring back at you and smiling. That's where lust lives—in that smile, in that look, in that tightening low in your belly that reminds you of how you started and why you go on, together.

SENSUAL SUGGESTIONS:
THIS IS IT

It's easy to be so wrapped up in the moment that you forget it can't last forever. Or can it? Make a promise to never forget the amazing desire for each other that first brought you together.

1. Keep a jar of memories. Throughout the year, write down your favorite romantic, sexy, tender moments. Reread them together whenever you need a reminder.

2. Make videos. Whether it's your version of a celebrity sex tape or singing a silly duet in the car, videos stand as reminders of the couple you are now—and the couple you always want to be.

3. Talk about the good stuff! Not only with your partner, but with your closest friends, too. Tell your love stories whenever the proper occasion presents itself. (Leave the juicy details to their imaginations, though!)

EROTIC FICTION

TAKE IT OFF

SOMMER MARSDEN

The first thing I said about my husband to my sister was, "He's not my type." Turns out I've never been more wrong in my life. Happily, happily wrong. What I was sensing so many years ago in this man was the fact that he was not selfish, childish, immature or, ya know, a jerk. All the things I was used to in the guys I was dating. It only took one date for me to see that he was kind and funny, super smart and so in tune with me from date one it was damn near scary. Seventeen years later and he's still so in tune with me it's damn near scary. And yes, every time we're together my stomach still does that funny thing where it feels like I'm falling. I think it might be because after all this time I'm still falling for him.

*I*t's silk and lace. The color of cream. It costs a fortune and I like the way it swishes though I'm not a girly-girl. Big occasions call for big gestures, at least that's how I suckered myself into buying this thing. It was a big purchase made with only a little thought. But after an expensive dinner and flowers, dancing and flirting, stolen kisses under streetlights and a few more for good measure on the drive home, a big dramatic reveal seemed...logical.

Though he prefers me naked. Always will, I'm pretty sure.

I come into the room feeling suddenly nervous, a bit silly, but a bit pretty, too.

He takes me in, his eyes flitting to all the places I want them to go. My breasts, crushed prettily to the soft bodice. The flare of my hips, pushing nicely against the silk to show off that yes—I am a woman, shaped like a woman, perhaps even more so than when we met. He holds a hand up to me and I suddenly feel shy and silly again, but fuck me, so sexy, too. But that's more because of his gaze on me than this fancy getup. My heart never fails to pound when we're together. My cheeks never fail to ignite with quickened blood.

"That's nice. Take it off." He curls his thick fingers in the cream-colored silk of my nightie and tugs.

Just like that a streak of excitement flares up the back of my neck, making my scalp tingle, my body shiver. I smile, moving away, teasing him with my body to say that maybe—just maybe this time—I won't obey. But I will, I always do. After all this time, when we're together my stomach drops as if I'm in freefall.

"Where you going?" James teases.

"I'm right here."

"Take it off," he growls again. This time his fingers travel up the thin lace straps that hold my gown up. I've dressed up just for our anniversary tonight, but deep down I knew what his response would be. What it always is.

That's nice. Take it off.

"In a minute." I slide my body along his, kissing his stubbled jaw, stroking my fingers over his chest, down his belly, a bit lower but not low enough to put my hands where I know he wants them. I can feel it radiating off him like heat—his want is palpable. It always is.

His fingers slide along the silken shield of the lingerie and he sighs. "It's so intrusive." Even as he tells me this, he's stroking my nipples to brisk attention. They tingle as the slide of silk adds an extra friction beneath his fingers.

"I know, baby," I say, skimming my tongue down his neck to nibble at his collarbone. His cock is hard under my hip and he moves just enough for me to feel it even more—want it even more. I'm not the only one who's teasing.

"Rita, what did I tell you seventeen years ago on our wedding night?" His voice is rough and deep and I can hear the desire there.

He's found the hem of my gown and is slowly, insistently, scooting it up over my knees, inching it up my thighs. My pulse pounds thick and heavy in my pussy and my stomach. I can feel it in my temple and my throat. I'd give a million dollars at this moment to have him touch me—make me come. If I had a dollar for every time I've felt this way, I might have close to that million, after all.

I try to distract him by rubbing against him, my breasts smashing the silk he dreads so much against his chest. My mouth brushes his, my tongue licking at his lips to make him want me even more.

He growls. I've succeeded.

He pins my wrists up by my breast and kisses me hard, trapping me to his chest even as my knees start to tremble from having to hold myself steady over him. His mouth is demanding, his breath staccato. He's still in boxers and I'm still in this ensemble I figured I'd put on just to celebrate another year together. What a silly thought that had been.

"You said take it off," I gasp, finally answering his question.

"'That's nice. Take it off,'" you said.

"That's right." He releases my hands and even as I cover him with my body, sliding against him to feel the hard planes of his angles against my softer curves, he grips the hem again, intent on sliding it up.

It slides above my ass and cool air kisses my skin. I gasp and give in. It's no use denying the fact that I want the damn thing off, too.

"And so now, seventeen years later, I'm asking you again to…" He cocks and eyebrow and stares at me. His big green eyes a bit shiny with lust. His mouth a kissable half-assed grin.

"Take it off?" I pretend to guess.

"Now," he says, and his hands are back on the hem tugging and this time I'm helping him. Of course I am.

That little slip of expensive fabric seems like a woolen dress as we wrestle and tug at it. It hits the floor with a whisper at the foot of the bed. He moves fast, pinning me under him, my thighs pressed wide by the bulk of his body, and a moan slips past my lips. This is always the best part. The part where the fucking is imminent, but my god, we have to get there first. Pinned under his big body, held captive by his warm lips, his eyes eating me up before he even touches me.

He catches that look and puts a finger—a gentle touch—to the center of my forehead. "What's going on in there?"

He's rotating his hips left to right, left to right, grinding his hard cock—still hidden beneath navy-blue boxers—to my thumping clitoris.

"Nothing," I lie, and then I laugh. I just made myself sound empty headed.

"Always something going on in there," he says, and finds me with his fingers.

His thumb sweeps over my clit even as he pushes a finger inside me and then a second. A shivery breath escapes me. He has me in the palm of his hand. Quite literally.

I try to keep my voice brave and steady as he begins a rhythmic pressure inside of me. Flex, release, flex, release. Every motion of his big hand sending signals to my body to get wetter, looser, tighter, wanting... My pulse picks up; the breath in my lungs is a heavy thing as pleasure sneaks closer and sits to wait for me.

"What did I say all those years ago about hand jobs?" I manage. I lick my lips and he follows with a kiss. His tongue is warm and soft and still tastes of fresh berries from our dessert.

Lips pressed against the pulse in my throat he says, "That hand jobs don't get you off."

He's added a third finger to my willing pussy. I seem to become liquid for him, adapting to whatever he wants to do, welcoming him with slick ripples of perfect physical joy. His thumb presses my clit once more and I am so close—almost there.

"And that was?" I sigh.

"A lie," he says, and laughs. I watch his serious face—he always studies me when he makes me come as if memorizing everything that brings me bliss. Three more hard, deep flexes of his thick fingers and I'm coming. The orgasm rushing toward me as soft and silken as that nightie we abandoned.

"A lie," I moan, riding out the ever-shifting waves of my peak. "A lie. But only for—"

"Only for me," James says, and kisses the place directly between my breasts. The place that gets damp with sweat when we fuck. He follows the kiss with a drag of his tongue and I watch him descend my body, strong hands clamped to my hip bones.

His face presses between my thighs, and I'm still so sensitive from coming I feel like I have a hair trigger. My thighs go tense around his face as he touches me with his tongue.

"Too sensitive, too sensitive," I chant, tightening up, trying to withdraw. I always do this—and he always knows better. You'd think

I'd learn. Or maybe I just don't want to.

He clamps his mouth over my nether lips, tongue gentle against my clit. It still feels like too much—much too much—at first. After just a moment, my body calms, warms to his wet ministrations and just like when his fingers were buried deep inside of me, I seem to bloom for him.

I always bloom for him. It's never failed to happen in all these years. Because of times like this—when it all comes down to nothing but us. Nothing in the whole world. Just for a bit.

My body's need to retreat becomes the exact opposite and everything unclenches, unfolds, and I am sprawled there on the bed, open to him, moving up to meet his gorgeous mouth with my body. His tongue is an ever-seeking, ever-surprising thing, licking at me in a way that makes me want to chase the pattern of its movements and yet there really is none to be found. So I surrender and within moments I'm coming again, arching up beneath him, so very happy that damn nightgown is gone. His fingers feather across the small jut of my hip bones, and I find myself laughing.

I always laugh when we're together. Laughter is the sound of happiness.

He glances up from between my legs, lips still dropping soft kisses on my inner thighs, and a thrill shoots through me. That look—that look that says, *I will take you and make you mine.* Though I already am. A hundred thousand times over...his.

The boxers come off, making a less subtle whisper as they hit the floor, and he's surging up over me, pushing my thighs wide with his body. I can't help myself, I move up under him, parting myself farther as he slides the smooth rigid tip of his cock to my slick entrance.

My want has become need, and I am mindless with it. No more talking. No more joking. He's sliding his glans along my pussy but not entering me. He drags it across the sensitive swell of my clitoris and I grip the bedsheets as if I'm dying and clutching them this way will save me.

"What did I tell you seventeen years ago, Rita?" He grins at me.

I lick my lips. I know the answer.

He enters me inch by slow inch—stretching me so lazily I feel like I might scream—both from pleasure and from frustration. And then he stays there, not seated fully, waiting for my answer.

My heart pounds hard enough that I can see the skin above it jumping. Jump-jump-jump as I toss my head and whisper.

"I love you."

James pushes deep this time, filling me all the way, the base of his cock slamming down on my eager clit. The power jolts through me hard, like an impact, before spreading out in sweet, syrupy waves beneath my skin.

I'm going to come again.

"And?" he asks, moving forward in intense but somehow idle thrusts.

"And it's still true," I answer.

"More than you know," he says, rotating his hips from side to side. All the invisible bells and whistles in my body that are really nerve endings and pleasure centers tell me it's coming, but I am still staggered with the force of it.

I am coming once again when his tempo speeds up as he gets close to doing the same. His rhythm is a delicious frantic dance of urgency. When he grows still for a heartbeat and our eyes lock, just as his orgasm hits him the hardest, I take his face in my hands and kiss him like it might be our last.

"Oh, I know. Because I feel it, too," I say against his lips, and I feel his release rush through him like a violent wave and I smile. Because I did that.

EROTIC FICTION

THE PROPOSAL

CHRISTOPHER COLE

I was a geek in college (who am I kidding? I'm still a geek) who knew a little about a lot of stuff, but I didn't really know much about women. They seemed to like me anyway, and I often found myself perplexed by that fact. Still, I never counted on getting married. I figured I'd end up alone, shuffling around my apartment in my bathrobe watching sports, writing about baseball and playing World of Warcraft. I imagined I would have a cat. A very macho cat. I do shuffle around the house in my bathrobe on the weekends, and I watch sports and play WoW and have a cat (and a dog), but I have this amazing woman with me to share it all. I'm not sure how I got so lucky, but I'm grateful she chose me.

*J*ust relax," she said.

I muttered, "Easy for you to say," but I tried to relax. It was a difficult task, seeing as how I was sprawled out naked except for a towel on the tiny bathroom floor and she was practically straddling me. Under other circumstances, I might have enjoyed it. In this case, it was awkward and embarrassing and I felt like an idiot. I was hoping the floor would open up and swallow me whole.

Megan, my girlfriend. I rolled the words around in my brain for a minute, tested them on my tongue. I couldn't get used to it. This beauty, with the long hair and dark eyes, aquiline nose and full, sensual mouth; she was my girlfriend. Me, who couldn't take a shower without slipping and falling and busting my head open on the counter as I was getting out.

"I'm a klutz," I groaned, as she efficiently treated my wound.

"Shut up," she said. "You need a rug in here."

I winced as she dabbed at the blood on my forehead. "Ouch. That hurts. Where did you get your nursing degree?"

"Shut up, it's barely a scratch. Don't be a baby." Megan is all about tough love.

"Yes, ma'am."

I watched her eyebrows arch. "Compliance? Really? You must have a concussion."

We'd been together-together for eight months. Before that, it had been a year of off-and-on dating while she finished graduate school and I got my post-grad-school feet wet at a dotcom startup. We hardly saw each other during those months—late-night dates for drinks, squeezing in time for coffee between her classes and teaching and my twelve-hour workdays. It was crazy, really, but even while I was opting to get up an hour earlier than normal just so I could meet her for a latte and a bagel, I realized I was falling in love. You know it's love when you're willing to give up sleep.

Yet here we were, eight months after we'd had the "I just want to be with you," conversation, with me bleeding on the tile floor and her biting her lip as she applied two Sesame Street bandages she had fished from the depths of her purse because I didn't own so much as a first-aid kit, and I just knew this was it. This was my future. Not the being on the floor bleeding part (though I'm embarrassed to say it wouldn't be the last time), but the woman, the feeling that I couldn't live without her, the love I felt for her, the erection that was tenting the towel around my waist despite the dull ache in my head. It wasn't perfect or neat or proper, it wasn't the time or place to be thinking what I was thinking, but it was ours.

"Marry me."

I don't think she heard me at first, intent as she was on blotting the blood that was trickling along my hairline. But then she paused and looked in my eyes. "Yes, you definitely have a concussion," she said.

"No, I don't. Marry me."

I could see the smile teasing the corners of her mouth. Was it a yes? Was it a maybe? It couldn't be a no—no woman would put up with my geeky idiosyncrasies and quirks unless she loved me. At least, I didn't think so. She was staring at me so hard that I was starting to wonder.

"Okay."

I blinked. Just like that we were engaged. "Okay?" I asked. "I propose and your response is 'okay'?"

She laughed and got to her feet. "Good point. It's clear you put a lot of thought and effort into your proposal. You even dressed for the occasion," she said, gesturing to my tented towel. "And you brought a friend."

"Fine, that's fair," I said, hauling my sorry ass up and groaning as my body protested my untimely fall. "But you said yes—or 'okay,' rather—so you can't take it back."

I nudged her out of the doorway and across the narrow hall to my bedroom. The bedroom was only slightly bigger than the bathroom, but at least there was a soft bed and no sharp edges for me to worry about. Gently pushing her back on the bed as she laughed at me, I was grateful she was the type who didn't care about a bed being made as long as we were making something else.

My towel was barely held in place by damp skin and a massive erection, so it didn't take more than a hip swivel to completely undo it and let it fall to the floor. She raised an eyebrow, but didn't say anything. Clearly, the ball was in my court and after my impromptu apology, I knew I had better make this good.

"So, about my proposal," I said, making quick work of undoing her jeans. "I have a few additional points to make before you give me your final decision."

"I already gave you my final decision." She shucked her top off, along with her bra. I paused for a moment to admire the sway of her breasts before continuing.

"Yes, but I want you to be absolutely, positively sure that it's your final, final decision. Until death us do part," I said solemnly. "This is some serious shit I'm talking about."

She giggled. "Uh-huh. If you say so."

I got her jeans down her legs, along with a pair of dark-blue panties that had a telltale wet spot in the crotch. That sort of derailed my thought process for a moment, but I pushed through. "I say so."

I knelt on the floor and spread her legs. "First of all, if you marry me, I can promise you that you will enjoy oral sex on a regular basis."

"I see. And how would you define 'regular'?" she asked, playing along. Only I wasn't playing—I was dead serious about wanting this woman to marry me and I wanted to give her the world for the rest of our lives.

"On demand."

She let out a long sigh. "Can't get more regular than that."

I licked up the inside of her leg, from the crease of her knee to that sweet, soft curve at the top of her thigh. Close, but not quite where she wanted me to be. I inhaled her scent—sweet, musky, enough to make a grown man cry.

"Exactly. And that's not all." I said it with the enthusiasm of an infomercial hawker. "There is so much more."

She squirmed on the bed, nudging me with a knee. She was impatient to have my tongue on her clit, I knew. And I knew exactly how she would respond when I finally gave her what she wanted. A quiet gasp, a sigh, her thigh muscles tightening and quivering as I licked her. I could hardly wait, but I did.

"What else?" she finally asked when it was clear I was in no hurry.

"Breakfast in bed on Sundays, chick flicks every Friday night and I will ignore the Johnny Depp calendar hanging in the bathroom."

"Mmm," she murmured. "Is that all?"

"Is that all? I think you need to pause for a moment and consider the beauty that is my French toast and the fact that I can't stand romcoms. Or Johnny Depp."

She giggled and I took that moment to lay the flat of my tongue against her clit. The giggle turned to that familiar gasp-sigh combo that still drives me nuts. When I made to move away, she put her hands on my head and guided me back down. I laughed, mouth open, tongue dipping into her pussy. She wriggled against me, hands tangled in my hair, as I began licking in earnest.

"Your French toast is a thing of beauty and so is Johnny Depp," she acquiesced with a grunt as she angled her hips up to meet my mouth. "But he's hardly as beautiful as you are right now."

That's my girl, a hopeless romantic who knows exactly the right thing to say.

I'm sure there were a couple of comments after that, though my hearing was muffled by the smoothness of her thighs and I'm not quite sure she could make out much of what I said with my mouth full of her sweetness. When her orgasm came, she arched off the bed like she'd been struck by lightning and all I could think was, *I did that. Me,* and I swear I could've come right there, without even touching myself, if she hadn't tugged me up by the hair just then.

"What else?" she gasped, using her hands and legs to pull me up along her body.

"Greedy wench."

She reached between us and finally touched me, wrapping my iron-hard cock in her hand and guiding me between her legs. "Yeah, I am. And right now I want *this*."

She was so warm and wet, so ready for me. I knew she would be, after that orgasm, but still—it never gets old, that feeling. She took me in, pulled me in, it felt like, until I was as deep inside her as I could go. She hitched her legs up high on my back so that I could feel every ripple of her pussy around me. I could barely think, much less talk, but the lady had asked me a question.

"Chinese takeout at midnight when you can't sleep," I whispered in her ear. "Doing your ironing because I know you hate it."

"You hate it, too!"

"But I love you," I said, though it was more of a groan as I couldn't take it anymore and had started to thrust. "And I want to spend my life with you."

"Okay," she said, gyrating her hips just so in a hula move that always lets me feel every millimeter of her. "What else?"

"You want more?"

"Oh yes," she whimpered, her pussy clenching down tight on my erection. "I want it all."

"You can have it, sweetheart," I said, meaning it in every way possible, but intent at that moment to give her—and me—an orgasm.

There wasn't any more talking for a few minutes, just her sighs and whimpers and my rather undignified bellow of pleasure when she stretched one leg down and hooked it around my calf while keeping the other one high on my shoulder. Her pussy seemed to narrow to a vise-like grip—a very orgasmic vise-like grip—and I lost all coherence, and possibly consciousness, for a few seconds. Somewhere in that void, I heard her own blissed-out cry. I was pretty lost in the sensations of the moment, but I did hear one thing clearly.

"Yes, oh god, yes!"

Once I regained the blood flow to my limbs and my cock had fallen into a state of sleepy satisfaction, I shifted off her and nudged us both around on the bed. With her nestled in my arm, damp hair strung out across my chest like a net I was very happy to have been caught in, I sighed.

"You said yes."

"I did not. I said 'okay.'"

"Nope," I argued. "That was definitely a resounding 'yes.'"

She laughed. "No woman cries out, 'okay, oh god, okay' when she's having an orgasm—not even an okay orgasm."

I tweaked her nipple. I couldn't resist. "So that was a 'yes' to the orgasm and not a 'yes' to my proposal of marriage?"

Her expression turned serious as she pressed a finger to the bandage on my forehead. I had completely forgotten what had led us to this moment. That's how good the sex was—and how in love I was.

"Yes, I'll marry you." There was no ambiguity there, no humor in her expression. She was serious. This was real. "But I want one more thing."

"Anything," I said, and I meant it. Then, and now.

"You have *got* to invest in a first-aid kit. You're a klutz."

TWO

BEYOND NEWLYWED LUST—
AFTER THE HONEYMOON

I guess I knew we couldn't sustain the level of sex we were having in those first few months, but I was surprised it dropped off so dramatically once we got settled into married life. Now it feels like we're expected to have sex whether we want to or not just so we don't fall into the rut of not having sex at all.

—Wendy, married three years

J very clearly remember the first night my husband and I *didn't* have sex after we got married. It was momentous because, up until then, we'd had sex every single day we were together. We'd been married almost three years at that point and had just moved from Virginia to South Carolina and bought our first house. It was a big deal. We were in our midtwenties and already homeowners! I felt like we were playing house and waited for someone to ring the doorbell and ask to speak to my mother.

Between moving, unpacking, painting, yard work and the other hundred tasks that are involved in setting up a household, we were having a blast, but we were exhausted. Most days, we found a way to squeeze in sex, even if it was a quickie. But after about a week and a half of being in that house together, working long days to get things done, we were starting to pluck at each other's nerves and neither of us had the energy for sex. I remember lying in bed that first sexless night, so tired my teeth hurt, thinking something was very, *very* wrong because we hadn't had sex. If I'd had one ounce of energy, I probably would've pounced on him and resolved the panic attack I was having. But I didn't have the energy to do more than worry about what it meant. I fell asleep, and we had sex the next morning. All was right in my world once more. Until it happened again a few days later.

I look back on those days of needless worry, and I have to laugh at how naïve I was. It took a while to realize that not having sex every single day didn't mean anything other than we were a normal couple with a lot going on in our lives. And before you write me an angry letter saying you don't want to hear about how we had sex every day for three years, let me add this caveat: I married a sailor in the U.S. Navy who was deployed more than he was home those first three years. In fact, he was gone nearly nine months of our first year of marriage, eight months the second year and six months the third year. So yes, we had a lot of sex when he was home, but it was always with the thought in the back of our heads that we'd be separated again soon. Deployment homecoming sex is a lot like honeymoon sex—exciting and new—and in our case, it was propelled by the external circumstances of having not seen each other in months.

Once we were together for an extended period of time and he had orders for shore duty and we had all the days we wanted to have sex…well, real life took over and our sex life slowed down a little. Routine, something that military families don't know a lot about, was a wonderful change of pace from deployments, training schedules and shift work. And, like most couples sooner or later, we hit that point in our relationship where our sex life dropped off. Not dramatically, but enough for me to notice and be concerned. These shifts vary for everyone and fluctuate like everything else in life; there are ebbs and flows to a healthy married sex life. There are times when it seems like you can't ever get enough and times when you're okay with going a day or two (or a week or two) without. There is no "normal" when it comes to your sex life. You can't compare yourself to friends (they lie) or magazine articles (they have their own agenda) or even studies that say couples have sex an average of X times a week. That X might as well be a question mark for reasons as varied as what I've stated above: people lie, they have their own agenda, they forget, they want to seem "normal" so they say what they think they're supposed to say or, most importantly, they're not *you* and it doesn't matter what they say.

How often you are having sex—and how often you *want* to be having sex—is only important to two people: you and your partner. And what happens behind closed doors, what is discussed or negotiated, what is shared and confessed, what is done in bed or what is only fantasized about, is absolutely, completely, one-hundred-percent normal. The only two people you have to please are your partner and yourself. So forget everyone else, forget what your best friend told you, forget about the studies and whether they appeared in *Cosmopolitan* or *The New York Times* or some academic journal with a longer subtitle than the *Cosmo* article, and focus on sharing yourself—*all* of yourself—with your partner.

Once the honeymoon period is over, couples tend to let out a long, slow breath and think that's it. They're settled, they're partnered, they can relax. And that's true—to a point. There is something to be said for finding The One and committing to a relationship for the long haul. But it's important to remember that whatever issues your brought into your marriage—whether you were aware of them at the time or not—are still there. In "Circuit," by Charlotte Stein, an inability to communicate about the most intimate aspects of sex creates a longing for more—a deeper bond. My story, "The Weight of Things," is about insecurities so many of us deal with—or don't deal with until someone we love shows us a different way of looking at ourselves. Though the situations are completely different, both stories share a common theme: the need to talk about your deepest fears, your wildest desires, the baggage you have carried alone until this point. It's scary, sure. Those words you can't or won't or don't say are terrifying to even think about. But once said—or written—they can make all the difference. *All* the difference.

If you had different attitudes about what was enough (and the right kind of) sex before you got married, those differences are still there. If you had body image issues or difficulties communicating or insecurities about your sexual performance—they're still there. It's *all* still there for both of you and you both will, at some point, have to confront it, deal with it and move beyond it. Because that's what a marriage is all about—working together and moving forward together. And a good lifelong sex life with your partner is one of those things that is absolutely worth working on and fighting for at every stage of your marriage, even while you're still on a honeymoon high and looking blissfully toward the future.

SENSUAL SUGGESTIONS:
KEEP IN TOUCH

Remember when you couldn't keep your hands off each other? Living together may take the edge off the need for the constant touch you experienced in the early years, but touch is still important.

1. Hold hands even if it isn't something you usually do. Always kiss each other good-bye, even if you're just running to the store. Curl up on the couch together when you watch a movie.

2. Enroll in a couple's massage class and rediscover each other in a new, therapeutic way. You can take what you've learned and explore the benefits of erotic massage in the bedroom.

3. Shower together whenever you can. It doesn't have to be about having sex (although there's nothing wrong with that!); it's about staying connected. Plus, getting clean now can lead to getting dirty later!

EROTIC FICTION

CIRCUIT

CHARLOTTE STEIN

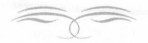

When my husband and I first started dating, I decided to do something very naughty. He knew I loved to write, so I thought I'd introduce him to some of my work in a very particular way—I would write him a filthy letter and leave it for him to find. And naturally when he found it, he'd be shocked by my daring. Maybe he'd even be stunned and appalled by the previously unknown depths of my filthy mind. I went to see him, filled with nerves, on the day after the letter had been delivered. I was terrified! I was sure our relationship was about to end! And then he said the words every girl longs to hear, after baring her perverted soul: "I couldn't read your handwriting." So I suppose the lesson is: never deliver your wildest fantasies in the incomprehensible scrawl of a maniac. Just do what I did, about thirty seconds later and after much amusement: I whispered them in his ear instead.

I can tell there's something he wants to say, even though he's not saying it. It's hovering around the edges of everything he does tell me, from *Please pass the peas* to *Maybe move a little to the left*. In fact, it's in that last one, in particular.

He means *Move all the way over to the left*, really. He means *Keep going until you touch me right there*, I think—but of course he can't quite bring himself to spell it out. He's my big, burly beast of a man; my blunderbuss who barreled me over. He stormed into my life at six foot five with shoulders like a milkmaid's yoke, and didn't give me chance to say no. Before I'd caught my breath we were married, and now here we are.

Caught between the image we have of each other—forceful, gorgeous, aggressive Tate and his petite and timid wife—and the seething reality. The furtive, delicious, reality. It's almost like I'm feeling all over him for his tender underbelly, and the farther I go with it the more excited I become.

By the time we get to our one-month anniversary, I'm desperate for it. I'm desperate to peel back his skin, to learn his secrets, and more than that—I'm desperate for him to share. He hadn't seemed so stoic and reserved when it came to sex, before. Our first fuck had been up against the cabinet in his office, him so unbearably assertive about it I'd climaxed before he'd completed his first thrust.

I like it when he's forceful. I like it when he comes through the door and has that look in his eye, and then he'll simply bend me over something and take me like that. Still too dazed to speak, body taut and trembling and unable to process the sensations he shoves through me.

Yeah, I like that all right.

But he has to know that I'd like him the other way, too—if that's what he's after. His hips jerk a little under my pressing hands and there's a hint of it, there's always a hint of it, and of course the hint gets stronger once he's almost let himself go.

Like when I suck him hard into my mouth and roll my tongue around the swollen head of his cock, just so. Yeah, he kind of forgets himself then, all right. Get him excited enough and the cracks will start to show...though that's both the problem and the solution.

Because there's only so long I can keep him like that. Push too hard and he'll just do it in my mouth, so overwhelmed by sudden filthiness that he can't quite keep himself in check. Hold back the slightest bit and he can go on forever and ever, expression as tight as a drum. Hands clenched into fists at his sides.

And then eventually he'll just haul me up into his arms and fuck me until I cry.

It's not what I'm aiming for. Or it is, it's just...marriage is supposed to be more, isn't it? You're supposed to learn and grow with someone, to share with them your deepest feelings and innermost thoughts.

And these are my deepest feelings and innermost thoughts:

That I want to, oh god, I want to do whatever he wants me to do. *Anything*, I think, *anything*, as I reach out one shaking hand and just sort of...pin him to the bed. Just a little, so that when I back away he can't buck up into my mouth.

Just enough that he knows what I've done, when he stops moaning and squirming and almost getting there.

He looks up at me—disorientated, I think. I've never shown him that I could be a tease, before, and it's unsettling for him, maybe. Or maybe it's the exact thing he's been wanting all this time, and that's why he stares down at me with that burning gaze.

He seems angry, I think. But there's something else amidst the anger. A kind of acceptance or a letting go, that gets stronger when I let him have one teasing lick, right over the curve of his tightly drawn-up balls. I cup his cock while I do it, too—just loosely—like I need to position him this way and that as I search out places to taste.

Which is almost shockingly exciting, in a way I can't explain. It buzzes through me, that near-indifferent handling of him; it makes me slick and warm between my legs. But a second after I've done it I know…it's not the thing he was after.

He's responding to me, but he's not going crazy. It's not quite the furtive secret beneath his many layers—though I suspect it's close. He likes to be teased, and he likes me holding him like this with my hand on his hip, and when I press down harder he likes it even more.

So maybe that's it.

Pain, I think, and then I shudder and shiver and don't know what to do with myself. Can I hurt him? Am I capable of something like that? He's so lovely, my husband, so open-faced and warm and safe. I don't want to carve a line into him and make him suddenly unstable.

Yet nothing feels quite as right as my nails digging into his skin, as he offers me a long, low moan.

"Oh, what are you doing?" he murmurs, but I think he knows all too well. I'm testing him out for weaknesses, and when I find one I exploit it mercilessly. I rake my nails down over his thighs and marvel at the way his head goes back. At the arch of that big, powerful body, now helpless.

But it's still not the one. He likes teasing, he likes pain—the secrets are coming thick and fast, now, and yet none of them is quite at his core. He wants something more, and the clue is in the tilt of his hips. That little entreaty he often offers me, to just go a little to the left, do a little more, touch me there, oh yes—

Between his eagerly spread thighs, I think, and then I rub one spit-slick finger down, down through that groove. That private groove that men don't like to talk about, in sexual terms—until you touch them there. Oh yeah, once you've touched them there they want to talk about it a whole lot.

"Oh god, I didn't know you could be so dirty," he tells me, in this one hot rush that sounds nothing like the him I knew before. This new guy is half-ashamed and half-excited, as giddy as I've never actually seen him. And more than that...

He's rubbing himself against my tentative, probing finger. He's urging me on in a way that makes it almost easy to just kind of ease inside him. Not a lot, you understand. Just a little way. Just enough to say:

I've penetrated my husband's clenching ass with the tip of my finger.

And he *loves* it.

Oh god, he loves it in a way I've never seen him love anything before, all overheated and too ready to come. His cock bobs against his belly, iron hard and so swollen at the tip. So red and slippery looking...ahh, yes. Yes, yes, yes, this is what I want. I want him wild and uncontrolled to the point where I can almost feel it myself. My pussy is one big pulsing hum, on the verge of an orgasm I shouldn't be able to experience without a hand on me.

But I think I'm going to. He's exposed some secret craving in me as much as I've exposed it in him, and now we're locked together like this, flushed with discovery. Mad with it. I think I'm going to burst, and the feeling only grows when he blurts out:

"Suck me while you do that. Suck me off."

So I do.

I take the head of his great, thick cock in my mouth, as I test the resistance between the cheeks of his ass. First the tip of my finger, then up to the knuckle, and finally all of it, twisting and turning inside his tight passage. It's completely smooth in a way I'd never imagined, and when I ease back and forth he clenches so tightly. He clenches around me and moans and bucks, and that deliciously hard cock pushes itself deeper into my mouth.

Of course the contrast drives me nuts. The give and take of it: me forcing my way into him and him doing the same in return. It's like we've made a loop, and every thrust and pull sends electricity surging around this closed circuit. I feel it crackle through my clit, my belly, my achingly empty cunt, and that's all I need.

I'm coming, I know. Or at least, I think. The sensation isn't of the usual sort, focused and spreading outward in one great wave. It tucks itself in tight, instead, and just kind of swells in on itself, not quite stopping when I want it to. There's a pain about it, a sense that I've not nearly had enough once it's done—but that's okay.

I'm not ready to end this yet. I need to see if he can do it, too—give himself over to something so completely that his orgasm seems almost apart from him. Like something forced on his body against his will, hard and fierce and leaving him desperate for more.

And judging by the sound he makes for me a second later—wrenching, guttural—I think I almost achieve it. I twist my finger just so inside him, searching out the one little spot that seems to make him half mad. Then just as I've found it I suck, hard, tongue lashing the underside of his swollen cock.

And the result is stunning. Overwhelming.

He doesn't so much come as go off, too hard for me to hold down. Every muscle in his body seems to stiffen all at once, but that's nowhere near the best part. The best part is the feel of his come spurting and spurting in my mouth, too fierce and thick for me to take. I can hardly swallow fast enough, hardly contain whatever this is—though I can't really say I want to.

I'd rather he break and burst at the seams like this. It's so much more satisfying than gingerly peeling back his layers, a bit a time. All of him just comes out all at once, in the feel of his cock spilling hard in my mouth and in the sound of his voice, as he shouts. I've never heard him be like this before or say the things he does:

"Yeah, yeah you little slut," he tells me, while I thrill over the rough *yeahs* and hum with pleasure over the *slut*. I'm not me anymore to him either, it seems. I can see it, now. I've not just ripped away his veil—

I've somehow shed my own, to reveal what I can be, underneath.

A whore. A desperate, greedy whore, who keeps swallowing his thick come and then returns for more. But even better than this is the look I see in his eyes, when I finally kneel up and face my big, sweet husband.

He doesn't mind.

Oh no, he doesn't mind *at all*.

EROTIC FICTION

THE WEIGHT OF THINGS

KRISTINA WRIGHT

When I was a high school freshman, I took a summer acting class with a young actor fresh from college and on his way to Hollywood. He was a family friend, and I had a tremendous crush on him. During our final evaluations, he told me that I was a competent actress (a glowing compliment to a starry-eyed fourteen-year-old), but I needed to either lose weight if I wanted to play a lead role or gain weight and play the "buddy" role. I remember my face freezing into a forced smile as I tried to mask my utter humiliation. I was neither skinny enough—nor fat enough—to be an actress? It wasn't a profession I aspired to; I had always wanted to be a writer, but to be told that my weight might interfere with a dream was upsetting to a young girl who believed she could, and would, accomplish whatever she set her heart on. I have never forgotten that conversation, but I am no longer embarrassed

by it or my body. I'm not an actress, true, but my happiness in life—including my sex life—has nothing to do with the size of my body and everything to do with the size of my heart, passion and imagination.

The lights are off. I am always careful to make sure the lights are off. Much like women become conditioned at an early age to suck in our stomachs when we stand up or minimize the amount of space we take up in a public place, I have conditioned myself to turn out the lights before I have sex. It's my version of foreplay. I need the darkness to allow myself to let go and free myself from the inhibitions of weight and imperfections and years of feeling inadequate because I did not look like the models in *Teen* or *Seventeen* or *Cosmopolitan*. I now know I don't need to be thin to be happy, but the need for darkness persists.

It is an illusion, this darkness. The blinds are open, light filters in from the streetlamp, from the nearly full moon, from the glow of the alarm clock announcing it's 12:25 A.M. I know he can see me—I can see him watching me. But the darkness gives me the illusion of invisibility. An illusion that allows me to feel beautiful, sensual, sexual, desired. Though I know he still wants me even in the light, it is darkness that frees me to be someone else—the real me. The darkness allows me to strut toward the bed, stripping off my T-shirt, then my panties, and climb on top of him. It is the darkness that allows me to guide him into me, one hand wrapped around his cock, the other braced against his chest. It is the darkness that gives me the power to lean down and whisper, "Fuck me. Hard."

But then—oh god—instead of putting his big hands on my big hips and fucking me, he leans over and turns on the bedside lamp. He is still firmly inside of me, one big hand is, in fact, anchoring me on him, but the other—the other is betraying me. Light, my nemesis, my Kryptonite, my worst fear, fills the room. Only, that's not true at all. It's a meager wattage beneath a thick linen-covered shade and the corners of the room remain cast in deep shadows. But here on the bed, in this place where I have shed my clothes and released my inhibitions, everything is illuminated. I am illuminated. He can see me.

"I want to watch you," he says, as if that forgives this unspoken breech of bedroom etiquette. "You're beautiful."

The compliment does nothing to ease the panic rising in me, overtaking the desire that moments ago had me hot and creamy with need. Now I feel cold and dry, a winter's night desert. I want to cover myself, but I don't even know what to cover. There is nothing I like about my body, not one thing. Except my hair. That, at least, is beautiful. And long. I stopped cutting my hair short years ago when an angry customer at the retail store I worked at referred to me as, "The fat girl." Now, at least, they say, "The girl with the long hair." I'm only "the fat girl" if someone asks, "Which one?"

All of this goes through my head as he is touching me. The imperfect breasts that are smaller than they should be, given the rest of my ample proportions. It's a cruel twist to be a curvy, Rubenesque woman and not have the breasts to match. But he touches them anyway, thumbing the nipples until they tighten, cupping them in his hands as if he loves them despite their imperfections. Then he has his hands on my waist and I feel myself willing my body to shrink, sucking in as hard as I can and still not being able to vanquish the roll that exists when I'm sitting down. He strokes down my sides as if it comforts him, as if testing the weight of me and finding it satisfactory. But I am still, still as a statue cast in marble, silently urging him to move on.

He slides his hands down my waist to my hips. I am a classic pear shape, my hips and ass carry the bulk of me. Men like my ass, they always have. It's an ass to hold on to, much more than a handful, and has a certain soft but firm quality about it that makes it fun to watch and more fun to touch (or so I've been told). I relax as he caresses my hips and moves his hands around to cup the globes of my ass. This is my comfort zone, or it would be, if only the lights were out. But no, he's still watching my every reaction as he spans my thighs and moves his hands up to the space below my round belly. Thumbs touch each other, then touch my swollen clit. I jump, my belly jiggles, and I'm torn between arousal and embarrassment. If ever there were a definition for the term *bittersweet,* this feeling is it.

"Relax," he says, as if reading my mind. And perhaps he is. He knows my insecurities, even if I don't talk about them. "Just enjoy how it feels."

"I can't enjoy it with you watching me."

I sound whiny. I *am* whiny. I have this amazing naked man inside me, rubbing my clit with the broad flats of his thumbs and staring at me like I'm some sort of decadent dessert, and I'm upset because there's a little light in the room. It's ridiculous and I know it. I know it, but I can't seem to stop thinking about the stretch marks and the dimples and the jiggle and roll of my ample body.

"What?" he asks so gently I think I might cry. This isn't how sex is supposed to go. It's supposed to be all hot, naked, *perfect* bodies and the only talk should be dirty talk. Right? But I take a deep breath and answer anyway.

"I'm fat."

"You're beautiful."

"I'm fat," I say, louder than I intend.

"I don't care how much you weigh," he says, and I know that to be true. "You are the most beautiful woman I've ever known, inside and out. And you're mine."

There's a little thrust that accompanies that last word that makes me let out a noise that's somewhere between a gasp and a squeak. It feels good.

"I can't relax when you're staring at me," I say again. "All I can think about is how fat I am."

"So close your eyes."

I stare at him. "That's not going to solve anything."

"I like looking at you, you don't like seeing that I'm looking at you. Close your eyes. Just feel it."

Then he does it again, a little thrust accompanied by his thumbs stroking along my engorged clit. And my eyes flutter closed of their own accord, because it just feels too damned good to keep them open.

"See?" he asks, sounding a little more self-satisfied than he has a right to be. "You feel amazing. And you look really hot when you're on top of me, by the way."

I growl in frustration and smack his chest. "Stop talking about how I look, or I'm not going to be able to come."

"Well, that is my goal, so I'll be good. Close your eyes again."

"You could just turn off the light."

He shakes his head, his expression turning serious. "Nope. I want to watch you. I want to see you move and feel you come and watch your skin flush and see every expression on your face from beginning to end. You are so beautiful."

It's hard to argue with an argument like that, so I don't bother. I just close my eyes. And while my self-consciousness is still there, teasing me like the faint lamplight taunts me from behind the creases of my eyelids, it's okay. I know he's watching—I even peek to see if he's closed his eyes, but no, they're wide open and watching me. Watching *me*. And I close my eyes quickly so he doesn't see me looking at him, but I feel something I haven't felt before. Empowered.

It's all still there. The extra weight that really isn't extra since it's been a part of me for as long as I can remember. The other flaws and imperfections, each one a reminder that I am not beautiful, not perfect, not one of those skinny girls I have envied since middle school. All of my imperfect and flawed parts are all still there, but somehow they're less worrisome. He's looking at me, naked, taking it all in. And he *likes* looking. He could close his eyes and imagine any one of a hundred Hollywood starlets or women he's known in the past—or the present. He could turn me into his fantasy, simply by closing his eyes and conjuring the perfect body. And yet…he's looking at me. Studying me. His eyes are fixed on my body, on top of him, riding him, pleasuring him. I *am* the fantasy. I am his fantasy.

It's as if a different kind of light comes on, one that kept me in a darkness of my own making. All this time, he's been telling me I'm beautiful, gorgeous, sexy—and I've tuned it out. The inner critic drowned him out. Muffled my own feelings of self-esteem and beauty. Maybe it's cultural; maybe it's the way I was raised to want to look like a standard of beauty I never understood, to be constantly on a diet—or feel guilty for not being on a diet, to suck it in and tighten it up through exercise or constricting undergarments that cost more than the outfit that covers them. Whatever it is, that little voice has been screaming at me louder than my own self-confidence.

And now, on the cusp of the kind of orgasm the poets write about, I'm having this epiphany that I am beautiful and gorgeous and sexy and absolutely worth looking at. And my eyes fly open as I realize— *so is he.* He is the most beautiful creature I've ever seen in my life, stretched out on the bed, muscles straining toward his own release. This is what I've wanted; this is who I've wanted. Always. Now. Right now.

I stare into his eyes, boldly, watching the way his face flushes as he tries to hold back, the vein throbbing in his forehead as he clenches his jaw to control his release. I swivel my hips—my big, beautiful hips—so that his cock touches every inch inside of me. I move his hands from my thighs, not to get him to stop touching me, but to move them up to my breasts. I cover his hands covering my breasts, squeezing him so he'll squeeze me. I moving faster now, my damp body slamming down on him and making wet noises as my pussy gushes around him. He's so hard and in me so deep it nearly hurts, but I want even that exquisite bit of torture. I want it all; I want him.

"Oh god, fuck me, baby," he says to me and I don't even flinch. I just stare at him as I ride him.

"Yes," I say. It is a yes to him, to fucking him like this, eyes wide open. It is a yes to myself to enjoy this moment, and every one that follows, because they are precious. It is a yes to this body of mine no matter what word I use to describe it—curvy, voluptuous, chubby, full-figured and, yes, even fat. "Yes, oh!"

The bed is squeaking and the headboard is bumping against the wall. I am hot, damp and ready, oblivious to anything but the feel of him inside of me and the tightening of my body that has nothing to do with sucking in my stomach or feeling tense. I'm there, right there, and then I'm free-falling. Or is this flying? Every muscle tightens, clamping down on him and the pleasure he is giving me. I'm gushing, soaking his groin and belly, rocking on him as he fills me with his own wetness. It's like swimming in the ocean when the air temperature matches the water temperature—my skin feels wet and dry, cool and hot. I'm splintering apart into diamonds, my eyes fluttering closed even while I try to keep them open and watch his every expression.

We're watching each other, serious, then smiling, then laughing, my body quivering with the need to release everything, feel everything. I collapse on top of him, burying my head in his neck and laughing great open-mouthed gasps of laughter. And then, my laughter turns into a sob and the tears are flowing even while I'm still coming, clinging to him as if he is the only solid thing in the room. And perhaps he is.

"What? What did I do?" he asks anxiously, pushing my hair from my face, trying to see me and hold me at the same time. "Did I hurt you? Oh god, I'm sorry."

Now I'm crying and laughing and trying to sit up even while it seems every muscle in my body has turned to liquid. "No, no," I giggle, gulping and trying to catch my breath. "I'm fine. I'm better than fine."

He doesn't believe me; his expression is so serious. "Then why are you crying?"

I can't explain it. There are no words. I swipe at my eyes, as wet as the rest of me, and smile. "I just realized how beautiful I am."

He opens his mouth to say something, though I can see from his expression he's not sure how to respond. But he studies my face and I'm still smiling, warm and flushed and happy, and he nods.

"You are," he says. "So beautiful."

I am. I really am.

THREE

GROWING YOUR LUST TOGETHER— NICE TO MEET YOU...AGAIN

The sex is still good and often enough to keep us both happy, but it still feels like something is missing, an intimacy that we used to share isn't there now. I know we aren't the same people we were when we got married, but I don't know how to tell her fantasies I've been having without sounding like I'm complaining or out of touch.

—Jared, married twelve years

$\mathcal{F}$antasy. The word is enough to give some people hives. If the idea of sharing your deepest, darkest sexual fantasies with your spouse sends you running into the closet, consider this: you got married because, in addition to being the love of your life and sexy as hell, this is the person you trust most in the world. Right? This is the person you trusted with your house key, the one you trusted to take care of you when you had that awful flu (hangover, broken leg, et cetera), the one you trust not to embarrass you in front of your friends, coworkers, parents. Trust is *hot*. It's sexy. It's one of the best reasons to get married. Trust and that peculiar way your beloved has of knowing exactly when to bring home chocolate or a six-pack or both.

Sharing your sexual fantasies is scary, sure. But the payoff is amazing. The payoff is intimacy like you've never experienced it. Yeah, I've also read the books and self-help articles that make it sound like all you have to do is tell your partner you want to be tied up and spanked with a spatula and you'll be having mind-blowing orgasms before you can say, "Ow!" and no, that's not really true. What's true is that sharing and acting out your fantasies is going to lead to fits of giggles and embarrassment and awkward positions (and, occasionally, moments of awkward silence) and pulled muscles that you won't be able to mention to your doctor without blushing. That's the truth.

So why do it? Well, here's the thing they don't tell you in the article about *69 Earthshaking Ways to Have Sex*—those fits of giggles and moments of embarrassment often bring you and your partner more intimacy than living out the actual fantasy. Seriously. People bond over things that make them uncomfortable, things that make them step outside their comfort zone. Think about your best friend in the world—and maybe it's the person you married—and what makes that person your best friend. Is it because you are always your absolute best, most attractive, most witty selves around each other? No, of course not. It's because you have seen each other at your absolute worst—you've done the most embarrassing things in the world in front of and with each other, you've confided things you wouldn't tell your therapist, pastor or mother. That's the difference between friends and *best* friends. And that is also what brings true intimacy in a marriage. The awkward moments, the inside jokes, the knowing looks. That's intimacy. Combine it with sexual fantasy and you have the makings of major fireworks (with laughter and eye rolling, too).

"Share your fantasies; take risks; be creative and shake things up a bit. Fun sex is about learning new tricks and experimenting, and meeting failed experiments (okay, maybe that whole duct tape and lollipop thing wasn't such a great idea) with giggles and kisses, not embarrassment and scorn," says Lori Bryant-Woolridge in her book *The Power of WOW.* "Playful sex also strengthens your intimate ties. Taking away the pressure of performance allows you to feel safer and more secure in your relationship, and this allows you to open up and communicate how you feel and what you want in bed."

Sharing your sexual fantasies isn't about being someone else— it's about being the person you want to be with the person you love most. Being your *truest* self. This kind of sharing is about honesty that you may not have experienced since you were dating. The truth is, most people are at their most honest early in a relationship when the stakes are still low. When your heart isn't involved and you can walk away at any time, you're likely to tell a partner anything. The longer we're with our partners, the more we inadvertently put up walls and barriers. But our interests and needs, including our sexual interests and needs, are not static; they change throughout our lifetime. And the person you should be opening up to about your interests and needs (in bed and otherwise) is the one you share every other aspect of your life with. The one who is going to be there through better or worse, richer and poorer, in sickness and in health—and through rug burns and misplaced sex toys, too.

Once you've been married for a while and settled into a routine, it can be difficult to open new doors. Complacency is a nice comfortable place to be—for a while—and then it can give way to boredom and frustration. If you're having a hard time getting the conversation started, try one of these:

• *"I had a dream last night..."* Leading with a dream scenario allows you to reveal every dirty detail of your fantasy without actually having to own up to it yet. You can gauge your partner's interest, open up the topic without too much embarrassment and explore it together in discussion before taking the leap to acting it out. There's a very real chance your partner has had the same "dream," but even if that's not the case, this approach works to introduce sexual fantasies that you may never have discussed before.

• *Keep a journal and share it with your partner.* Write your sexual fantasies as letters to your partner or as short stories, using the stories in this book for inspiration. You can use a traditional journal or send them through email. The very first erotic stories I ever wrote were in a leather-bound blank book that I gave to my husband when he returned from a six-month deployment. No one has—or ever will—read them but him, and that's the point. You don't have to be a professional writer and no one will see your words except the person they're intended for. For some people, reading (or writing) about sex is a little easier than talking about it. If your partner is enthusiastic about the idea, you could take turns writing letters or fantasies to each other.

• *Start your own erotic book and film club.* Take turns recommending erotic stories and movies. Buy two copies of a novel or anthology and read together in bed, discussing favorite stories or scenes. (The stories in this book are a great springboard for sharing erotica.) Watch an erotic movie together and agree to act out one scene from the film.

Communication is hot—*very hot*—as Jeremy Edwards demonstrates in "Communication Exercises." Opening up to your partner about a sensitive subject can lead to some very sexy fantasy sharing as well as a deeper sense of intimacy. But sharing your sexual fantasies can feel daunting when your day-to-day life is packed with career, family and household chores. Saying, "Hey, baby, I know I said I'd never do it, but I think I'm ready to try bondage. Please pass the broccoli," at dinner is a little abrupt and maybe not the best time to start the conversation. If the words don't come easily (or at all), don't give up. Find another way to share your fantasies. In "Bound for the Bedroom" by Christine d'Abo, it's a book that opens the door to communication and living out a fantasy.

It doesn't matter *how* you communicate, just that you do. Whether it's a conversation, email, book, film or something else, take a chance and get the conversation going. Do what works for you. It's your marriage; it's your sex life. This is your partner you're sharing your fantasies with, the person you love and trust most. Remember that and repeat it as necessary even if you're blushing and stumbling over the words as you go. And please pass the broccoli.

SENSUAL SUGGESTIONS:
MAKE IT CURRENT

Never forget the passion that brought you together, but remember that you both are ever evolving sexual creatures. Keep learning about the person you're married to.

1. Create a sexual bucket list together and talk about it—and any new interests—as you work your way through it.

2. Make out like you used to. Even if you went to bed on the second date, at some point you made out like fools because you weren't yet having sex (or didn't have a convenient place to do it). Do it again—and rediscover the joys of first base.

3. Take the *Cosmo* (or the magazine of your choice) sex quiz—but take it for each other. Answer the questions as your partner and see how well you know each other right now. Act out any questions you get wrong.

EROTIC FICTION

COMMUNICATION EXERCISES

JEREMY EDWARDS

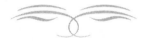

In the first ten or fifteen years of my adult life, there were several pieces of my identity as a sexual being that I had to learn to embrace rather than ignore. One of these was my internal responsiveness to the beauty or sexiness of some of the women I encountered in the normal course of events. My wife and I have been together—very, very together—as a couple since college days; and since ours is a monogamous relationship, this means the attractions of others have been moot (for lack of a better word) for practically our entire adult lifetime. But with the help of my wife's wisdom, trust and understanding, I learned that it was still okay to feel the way sexy friends and strangers make me feel, and to acknowledge—and enjoy!— those feelings. And the same goes for her, of course. We both recognize that getting a little tingle from a friend or stranger's eyes, laugh, legs or ass is one of the joys that enriches our lives.

I'm normally so direct, especially with Melanie. *Communication* is one of the preeminent watchwords of our marriage, and I'm a person who's naturally candid to begin with. By the same token, I'd developed the instinct, even with Melanie, to step delicately—not evasively, just gingerly—when a topic seemed potentially sensitive. And this seemed potentially sensitive.

And yet it was also important, I'd decided. We'd been together for four years now—married for three—and during that time I had consistently opted not to mention it when I found another woman's looks pleasing. You know: the sister of a close friend, who was visiting one weekend…that woman who waited on us at the Mexican restaurant…the female lead in the old movie we saw half of on TV one night. I would think it, but not say it.

Sometimes I'd think it again later and still not say it.

By contrast, I always spoke up if I'd thought the friend's sister was impressively smart, or the restaurant server delightfully friendly or the actress particularly funny. Eventually, the contrast felt unsettling—in the context of our no-secrets relationship, the self-censorship bothered me. Sure, there were things I kept to myself if they were trivial and gratuitously *negative*: no need to make a point of informing Melanie if I thought she'd been less effective than usual in that last round of charades, for instance. But thinking someone was pretty wasn't negative—was it?

We were secure. We were monogamous, but not jealous. We both, presumably, knew that being committed, even being committed forever and ever, didn't make you oblivious to the charms of the people around you. I was sure there were guys other than yours truly whose looks made Melanie think, *Ooh, very nice,* and I had no problem with that. I had to assume she wouldn't have a problem with the equivalent response in me. And though it wasn't specifically important that I happened to think the friend's sister was pretty or the actress was cute, I came to believe it *was* important, in a general way, that I not feel obliged to keep those reactions hidden from the love of my life.

Still, I wanted to broach this subject delicately. I didn't *think* it would be like Melanie to feel hurt or sad because I thought someone else was pretty or even beautiful; but people's emotions can be surprising sometimes. I was certain she wouldn't be bothered by it intellectually—she wouldn't think it wrong of me or consider herself betrayed or let down by it—but I couldn't entirely rule out the possibility that it might make her feel just a little awkward or put off. Though I was fairly confident nothing like that would happen, I tried to proceed carefully.

"That was a great party last night."

"Yeah!" said Melanie, with her characteristic enthusiasm. "I had a lot of fun."

"I'm glad. I particularly liked talking to Meg's friend Emily."

"Emily... Oh, right, in the paisley blouse. Yeah, me too. I really liked her."

"Very smart and funny and cool," I continued.

"Yeah."

Here it came. "I, uh, also thought she was quite beautiful."

I didn't see any sign that the remark shocked Melanie.

"I can see that, yeah. She has those high cheekbones and those big, expressive eyes."

There was tension in the room—but I judged it was all coming from my end of the love seat. Everything seemed to be going smoothly, yet still I felt nervous and stilted in a way that was rare.

I touched my wife's shoulder. "Hey...I hope it's okay for me to mention finding somebody beautiful." Was I actually trembling a little?

She put down the book she'd been leafing through, and beamed up at me. "Of course." As usual, she was a picture of even-keeled, easygoing benevolence.

"It doesn't make you feel threatened or neglected, right? You know it doesn't mean I'm any less in love with you—how wonderful you are, how beautiful you are, how much I…"

She cut me off, for the purpose of reassuring me that much sooner. "Of *course* not, Lawrence. Don't worry. I think it's perfectly normal for you to respond that way sometimes to other women. I would never have assumed you didn't."

"Oh, Mel, I love you. Thank you," I said earnestly.

"Also," she continued after receiving my kiss, "I'm always interested in hearing *which* women, whenever you want to share."

"Really? You're not saying that to humor me?"

She laughed. "No, I'm not humoring you." She poked me in the gut. "I'm genuinely interested."

I hugged her. "You're just…the best," I said. "And likewise—feel free to tell me when you think a guy is gorgeous, okay?"

"It's a deal." She gave me one of her playful little mock-businesslike handshakes.

But in my mind, there was one more loose end.

"And…all right, we're talking about finding somebody pretty, or beautiful—you know, *good-looking.* But what about finding someone…uh…*sexy?* Do you still think that's okay?"

She smiled indulgently. "Yes, Lawrence, sexy is okay. Hey, sometimes someone is just sexy to you—or to me—right? It's just part of being alive and aware. We're sexual beings, after all."

"That's how I feel about it, too," I said. "I'm very glad you agree—seeing as how you're my favorite 'sexual being.'"

"Mmm." She kissed me. "So, did you think Emily was sexy?"

I nodded. "There was something about her personality—and maybe her manner?—that I found…well, sexually attractive. Maybe part of it is the eyes, like you said. Not just their size and color, but the *way* her eyes look at you when you talk to her. What did you call them?"

"Expressive."

It was then that I noticed Melanie had a hand down her shorts.

"Hi," I said, waggling my eyebrows. This was how we typically initiated sexual frolics.

"Hi."

Daytime sex was uncommon for us, but not unheard of. With the sun streaming in sensually through translucent curtains and my wife's fingers pressed to her crotch, I couldn't imagine spending the next chunk of this summer Saturday afternoon any other way.

I took hold of Melanie's pants-plunging arm. "It's a stimulating topic, isn't it?" I gave a slight tug on her wrist, encouraging the activity of her fingers in her underwear.

"I admit I do feel a bit 'stimulated.'"

"Yeah, the hand in your pants sort of tipped me off."

Her free hand darted to the ridge in my jeans. "I have not yet begun to 'tip you off.' That will require a hand in *your* pants, my friend. But first, you'll have to unzip this."

As I did so, she moved in closer and whispered in my ear. "Fuck, it makes me hot to hear you talking about how sexy someone is. I'm a fly on the wall now at that party, watching while Emily makes you tingle."

She pulled her face back and kept speaking, at normal volume now but with just as much passion. "Did you start to get *hard* while she was talking to you?"

"Not exactly, but—"

"Oh, what the fuck, it doesn't matter. I'm going to imagine that she made you hard, regardless. I'm going to imagine that she made you as hard as...*this*."

"*This*" referred to the near-vertical erection that was thriving in Melanie's fist.

I deemed this a good juncture to make a bid for *her* juncture. So I yanked her hand out of her shorts, sucked briefly on the slightly sticky fingers and quickly sought the place they'd come from with my own fingers. She sighed when I touched her pussy lips.

For a minute or two we masturbated each other wordlessly, getting into the zone and grooving in a slowish—but not sluggish—tempo.

Then she resumed the conversation, without breaking the physical rhythm. "Speaking of all this stuff…"

Now it was Melanie who looked a bit nervous, as she prepared to launch into whatever confession our discussion had triggered. I took her hand and gave her my most supportive—and engaged—attention.

"There's—okay—there's, um, a young guy who waits on me sometimes at the convenience store near work." She hesitated, letting this beginning linger in the air while we stroked each other.

"Uh-huh?" I prompted.

"So…he's in his early twenties, I guess—clean-shaven, handsome guy with a sparkle. He always teases me about buying two yogurts at a time—never one, never three." The phrase *two yogurts*, as it happened, drew my gaze to Melanie's tightly T-shirted chest.

Having found her narrative, she seemed to relax, and the words flowed liquidly, as if lubricated by the slickness I was sampling with my fingers, between her legs.

"I'm a sucker for men who are kind but mischievous. Well, like you," she added with an affectionate grin. "This fellow has that vibe, and he's tall and skinny and looks like he could be the lead in some offbeat romantic comedy."

"And you think he's hot?"

Melanie laughed. "It's amazing how well you can read my mind, with the merest of hints."

I squeezed her, while managing not to lose contact with her pussy, or pull my cock out of her grasp. And I could see what she'd meant earlier about being "genuinely interested" in which women got my attention. It was one more facet of me—one more sexual facet—for her to share, as I was enjoying the privilege of being shared with in turn. It was definitely a thrill, I was learning, to hear about my wife having a sexual response to someone.

What better thing to share with one's lover, I reflected, than the specifics not only of what, but of *who* sparked one's libido? And why hadn't I come to that perspective years ago?

"The young rascal from the convenience store, huh?" I could understand why Melanie was attracted, given her description of his personality and appearance. Moreover, I don't think I'd ever actually used the word *rascal* before—so this dialogue was not only exercising our sexual-communication muscles, but expanding my active vocabulary as well.

The rhythmic motion of Melanie's hips became more emphatic; she was starting to squirm her way up the steep slope to orgasm. "Talk to me more about Emily now," she said in a soft voice.

I heard my own voice creep into the upper portion of my register, as her action on my dick ramped up in urgency. "Well…when I was lying in bed this morning, I was visualizing Emily's breasts. She's built small, remember, with petite breasts."

"True."

"But even though they're small, they're still *breasts*, right? I mean, they're sensitive—erogenous."

"Yes." Melanie was reflexively palming one of her own, more substantial, breasts while she listened.

"And it was turning me on just to consider that."

"Uh-huh."

"Her breasts, though they're small, aren't any less *intimate*. She—

she wears clothing over them, until she strips off her top to offer them to somebody...her sensitive, erogenous little breasts...intimately... with the nipples peaking and...oh god, Mel..."

"Go on, Lawrence—*please.*"

I struggled to continue speaking. "And...you know...although Emily's breasts are diminu—oh, fuck—*diminutive*...if someone touches one of her nipples—haha, like *this*—she—ahh—she feels the...electricity in her...in her cl-clit."

"Ahh!" Melanie writhed sinuously as I twisted her nipple.

And then we were coming, Melanie creaming in her shorts as my fingers raced back and forth from lips to clit; and I, spurting arcs of excitement where she clenched me, my pelvis convulsing with joy.

From that day on, we made a point of telling each other. It was funny how after having not mentioned such things for so long, we skipped straight to *definitely* mentioning them, leapfrogging right over the middle ground of *maybe* mentioning. But it made perfect sense: not only was it one more area in which to nurture our intimacy with communication; these particular exercises in communication also stoked our desire for each other. They made Melanie even sexier to me, and me even sexier to her.

And we realized that as foreplay, these revelations needn't stop at "he/she is like this and I think he/she is attractive." From Emily with her nipples exposed to the convenience-store dude jerking off over magazines in the back room, full-fledged fantasies about sexy friends, acquaintances and strangers were game for sharing as well....

"Would you like to hear my new favorite fantasy about that guy Terry?"

As always, I answered yes.

"It started when I saw him with a woman today."

"Wait a sec, Mel—refresh my memory. Terry?"

"Um-hmm. He's the one I told you about from the bike shop, with the red beard and the assortment of hats."

"Oh, right, I remember. The one who reminds you of a young Peter Ustinov who's been working out."

Melanie chuckled, and squeezed my balls under the covers. "I believe those were my exact words. I love how attentive you are."

I grinned modestly. "And you saw him with a woman today…"

"They were coming out of the café at lunchtime, and Terry and I smiled hello in passing. She seemed like a girlfriend—they were sort of squished together when they passed me. I can't swear his hand was on her ass…"

"I'll settle for ninety-percent certainty."

"So all afternoon, I was having these little fantasies about Terry and his perky blonde girlfriend."

"Such as?"

"Such as imagining that Terry lives upstairs from us."

"Uh-huh."

"I imagine we have our door open one night, and we catch a glimpse of Terry and his friend on their way up. She's flushed and giggling, in a flirty skirt—she's leading the way, though it's his place…having him chase her flirty-skirt ass up the stairs."

"Mmm."

"His body is godlike, and I can see his cock is hard. Very."

She licked her lips.

"And…in the moment they scamper by, I can tell the girlfriend is giddy with that unmistakable aura of *We've been drinking a little, and now we're going to fuck.*"

"Wow," I said.

She started grinding herself against me. "And then I imagine them upstairs—she sprawls backward onto a futon, say, with her legs wide open. The panties, if there ever were any, are gone, daddy, gone"— Melanie chortled with a manic horniness—"and Terry's spicy, masculine warmth closes in to fuck me."

I laughed when the pronoun hit my ears.

"Oh! I mean fuck *her*. Ha. I guess I got carried away." She was still grinding.

"Personally, I liked the sound of it when you said 'fuck *me*.'"

Her paws were all over my torso, her voice urgent. "Well, don't just lie there liking the sound of it, Lawrence…"

EROTIC FICTION

BOUND FOR THE BEDROOM

CHRISTINE D'ABO

I'm very fortunate to be able to say that I'm married to my best friend. I know not everyone is lucky enough to have that type of connection with his or her partner. The advantage for me is that even after being together for twenty-plus years, I can try out new things in the bedroom and not once have to question how my husband is going to react. I trust him implicitly to know exactly how much is enough for me. It can lead to some interesting times.

I'm not sure who was more surprised when I handed my husband the *How-To Introduce BDSM into Your Relationship* book: me, or my husband. I know it was not something he ever thought I'd be into, despite my enjoying the occasional slap, and the way I jump to do whatever he wants if he uses a particular tone in the bedroom.

I honestly never thought I'd get up the nerve to tell him. *Hey, sweetie, I don't mind at all if you want to tie me to the bed and pinch my nipples until I come. Oh, and can you flog me until I'm begging? Thanks!* It'd be kind of a hard conversation to approach after ten years of a happy marriage.

So as I was standing there, letting him read the back cover of the book, I desperately wanted to know what he was thinking. The kids were going to camp for the weekend, which would give us enough time and space to see where we might be able to take this. Worst case, I figured we'd at least be able to talk things over and maybe have sex on the kitchen counter. Best case, I'd be able to live out a few of my deeper fantasies. Either way, I wanted to give him time to mull it over. I'd learned long ago that he didn't like to have things sprung on him.

He quirked an eyebrow over the top of the book, his gaze traveling down my body as if seeing me for the first time. "Something you're trying to tell me?"

"I'd like to give some of this a shot." Of course he was going to make me spell it out. He was naturally dominant that way. "This weekend."

He nodded and opened the book to a random page. "Anything in particular?"

"I flagged a few things of interest." There was no way I was touching the book again. I'd managed to put the ball in his court, and I wasn't brave enough to take it back. "Just read it over and let me know what you think."

The kids came into the room then, looking for food and needing help with homework, cutting short any more conversation on the subject. He disappeared for a few minutes and when he came back the book was gone.

I don't know what I was expecting to happen, or when I thought it might occur, but I thought at least whatever *it* was, I wouldn't have to wait too long.

Friday night passed normally enough. We'd dropped the kids off at the bus that would take them into the wilderness for the weekend, came home and watched TV, and had sex before going to bed. Nothing crazy. He didn't tie me up and flog me. We had normal, comfortable sex. I came twice that night, but somehow I was still disappointed. Not that I told him that. I did come *twice* after all.

He disappeared early on Saturday morning. We normally went to the market and picked up our meat and veggies for the week. Sometimes, I'd get a box full of apple fritters too.

Left on my own, I puttered around the house, cleaning and making soup. I was just putting everything into containers to freeze when the garage door opened and closed. He came inside, arms full of bags.

"Did you get anything good?" I returned my attention to the soup. "Any treats for me?"

"Oh, one or two."

I wasn't paying attention as he put the groceries away. I don't even remember if we spoke at all, enjoying the unusual silence of our house. It wasn't until a silver bag was set directly in front of me, covering my hands and the sealed soup container, that I looked up at him.

"What's this?"

He gently bit the side of my neck. "Your treat."

So it wasn't apple fritters. I reached in and pulled out a stiff plastic package: a half-naked woman on the front was suspended by her hands and her feet. Velcro restraints.

Oh.

He leaned in and nipped at my earlobe. "I want you to go upstairs right now and get naked. Stand at the foot of the bed."

Oh. *Yes.*

I think I ran. I don't remember exactly, but I'm certain I was naked in less than three seconds. The room was cold, making my nipples hard. Goose bumps covered my skin. I wasn't nervous exactly, but the anticipation of not knowing what he planned was making me squirm. I settled for locking my hands behind my back and dropping my gaze to the floor. I was pretty sure that's what submissives were supposed to do. At least in all the books I read.

I'm not sure how much time passed before I finally heard his steps on the stairs. I didn't dare look up, though I desperately wanted to see the look on his face when he came in. I was certain he would enjoy this as much as I knew I would. He loved taking control in the bedroom, flipping my body this way and that while we had sex, though this would be different.

He stayed in the doorway and I could feel his gaze taking in my body. "There are a few things I think we need to talk about first."

My lips were dry, but I fought the urge to lick them. "Okay."

"I read the book. There's a lot of stuff in there I'm not sure I'll be comfortable with." My disappointment probably showed on my face, because he quickly stepped up to my side. "I'm not ready for that yet. But I did make a list of a few things I think we could start with. If it works for both of us, then we'll see where it leads."

I did look up then. My heart was pounding and I needed him to know how badly I wanted this. "I'll do anything you want."

He cupped my cheek. "I just don't want to hurt you."

"That's part of the point."

"When we got married I promised you I'd never do anything that would cause you pain. I'll do this if it's what you want, but there are lines I'm just not comfortable crossing. I love you too much for that."

"It's no good if both of us aren't into it."

It was his turn to grin. "Oh, I'm going to enjoy what I have in store for you. Just none of the crazy intense stuff. Not until we learn a bit more. Okay?"

"Deal."

"Good." I didn't suspect the slap to my bare ass, and cried out even as the burn spread across my cheeks. "Now, facedown on the bed."

The duvet cover was soft and quickly warmed by my body heat. I turned my face to watch him move about the room, securing the straps he'd bought to the legs of the bed. He tossed the loose ends up so they reached my body. I offered no resistance, smiling when he finally placed my wrists and ankles into the Velcro cuffs, securing me in place.

I tested out the restraints, squirming this way and that. I really couldn't move far at all and for a few seconds an overwhelming feeling of panic slammed into me. I couldn't get away even if I wanted to. I was completely dependent on my husband to set me free.

He sat down on the bed beside me and began to stroke my hair to calm my nerves. "I love you."

"I love you too." I let out a shaky breath. "Now what?"

"Are you comfortable? They're not too tight, right?"

"I'm good."

"Can't get away?"

"Nope."

"So if I do this, you just have to lie there and take it?"

A gentle caress trailed down my back. I bucked my hips, trying to increase the force of the light touch, but to no avail. Before I could even get my mind around that sensation, he smacked something hard and fast against my ass, sending a sting through my body and into my pussy. I groaned, enjoying the contrast. "What is that?"

He dangled the plastic spaghetti claw in front of my face. "We'll buy a new one."

Damn right we were. That wasn't leaving this bedroom. "Again, please."

Without warning, he pushed two fingers into my pussy, pumping me as he spanked my ass with the claw. The burning was offset by surges of pleasure that spread out from my cunt and into the rest of my body. I tried to buck my hips, pushing up into the slap, wanting to feel that sharp sting, surprised at how much I liked it.

When things were about to get too intense, he pulled back, flipping the claw around and raking the points down my back. It was almost too gentle, too much of a contrast from the spanking. I didn't know if I wanted to get closer to it or farther away.

We went on like that, mixing the sensations, gentle and hard, until my mind began to drift and all I could do was feel.

The next time he pushed his fingers into my body, I knew I wouldn't be able to hold back my orgasm. I groaned into the mattress and bucked in time with his fingers. He teased my clit with his thumb, pressing and grinding it until I lost control. I came with a scream, fucking myself back on his hand.

My mind was still buzzing as he pulled away, moving to my feet to free them. My hands were left as they were, but now he was able to pull my hips up. With one smooth push, he buried his cock full inside me.

"Oh fuck," he muttered. His fingers dug into my hips and he held himself still. "Your muscles are freaking out in there."

I couldn't formulate a response to that, so instead I pushed back against his cock, needing him to fuck me. He seemed to take the hint, increased his grip on me and slammed forward. With my arms spread out as they were, my face was pushed into the mattress. There was nothing I could do to stop him from doing whatever he wanted with my body. I trusted him more than any other person in the world, and I knew he'd never betray that trust. I was owned, cherished, his.

The dig of his nails in my hips was the only warning I got before he slammed hard into me and came. His guttural cry was a pleasure spike right through me, setting off another orgasm. I clung to the restraints and gasped for air against the fabric.

I think I might have passed out. The next thing I knew I was wrapped up in his arms. My ass stung. Not too painfully, though, and the rest of my body still tingled.

"Hey." He pressed a kiss to my temple. "So that was fun."

"Oh yeah." I snuggled in closer, enjoying the sound of his heartbeat against my ear. "Not bad for a first try."

His finger trailed down my back, stopping well short of my ass. "I didn't hurt you too much, did I?"

"I'm good." Nipping at his chest, I growled softly. "I liked it."

"I did too."

We'd been together long enough that I knew he had something else he wanted to say, but he didn't want to upset me. "What?"

"Don't take this the wrong way."

I rolled my eyes. "What?"

"Have you always wanted this? To be dominated?"

It wasn't as easy a question to answer as he probably assumed. "Not really. Maybe? It's not something I thought about to be honest. But I always love it when you take control and get all bossy. I love the slaps to my ass when I'm doing something. Only recently did I think there might be something more to it than that. So, I started reading."

"Gotcha." He scratched his nails along my arm. "Well, if you're open to it, there are a few things that I might like to try."

A shiver of lust went straight through me. "I think you might be able to persuade me."

"Good, because the kids are gone for another day and a half and I have a list."

We managed to try out most of those things.

The challenge has been keeping the kids from wondering what has happened to all of the kitchen utensils.

FOUR

LUST AFTER PARENTHOOD— PREGNANCY, BABIES AND TODDLERS, OH MY!

Our sex life was great for a few years after we got married. Then we had three kids in five years and things slowed down. Waaaay down. I feel like I shouldn't complain because we're still having sex (which is a nice surprise, since everyone told me when I was pregnant with our third that our sex life would be over now), but it isn't even close in terms of quantity or quality. I miss what we had.

—Kerry, married ten years

𝒯he most frequent comment I heard when I was pregnant with my oldest son was that my sex life was *over*. O-V-E-R. Even strangers felt compelled to tell me, "Things are going to change forever, if you know what I mean." *Wink, wink.* (These were often the same people who would attempt to touch my watermelon-sized belly without asking permission.) Interestingly, I somehow found enough time to have sex and get pregnant again when my baby was a year old, so I guess my sex life wasn't *over*. I don't intend to keep having babies just to prove that sex doesn't stop once you become a parent, so you'll just have to trust me on this.

But there are some realities when it comes to sex and becoming parents. Bad news first: having babies absolutely changes your sex life. Your friends, mother-in-law and the barista at Starbucks are telling the truth about that.

There are very real reasons why your sex life may drop off during pregnancy or in the first few months (or even years) after having a baby:

- *Your sex drive may decrease.* Hormones and exhaustion take their toll on you during pregnancy and in those first months (sometimes years) after you have a baby. And it's not just women who are affected. A recent study concluded that a man's testosterone level drops after he becomes a father. So there is a very real possibility that neither of you will want sex. And that's okay.

- *Spontaneity goes out the window.* Once you have a little one (or more) in the house, the days of going at it on the kitchen floor while dinner burns on the stove are generally behind you.

- *You might not want to be touched.* Having a baby or toddler clinging to you all the time can make you overly sensitive to touch. So even when the touch you're receiving is very much desired emotionally, your body simply may not enjoy it physically.

- *Your expectations might change.* You may both have been on the same page before you had kids, but things can change once you become parents. If one of you has unrealistic expectations of what your sex life will be once you're parents (either expecting more or less than your partner), it can really mess with your new reality.

- *Your schedules may not be conducive to sex.* If one of you is taking the night shift, or you work opposite shifts in order to save on childcare expenses, you might not see each other very much. It's hard to work sex into the schedule when one of you is always gone or asleep.

Every couple is different, but some or all of these may apply to you. (And if none of them apply to you, I'd really like to meet you!) Or there might be other reasons your sex life drops off, such as a relative staying with you for an extended time frame, body image issues post-pregnancy, stress and conflicts about parenting, et cetera. For whatever reason, *most* couples have less sex once a baby arrives on the scene. The good news is you mostly won't care. Does that not sound like good news? Trust me, it is. You will only have eyes for baby—at least for a little while—and your "little while" can range from a few weeks to a few months to a few years. Once the dust settles and you've had time to get your bearings as parents, you will look at each other and wonder who that stranger is sitting across from you. And because your "little while" might not be your spouse's "little while," it's important that you discuss your needs with each other. Like every other stage of marriage, communication is absolutely key to thriving as a sexual couple during the tough and exhausting early parenting years.

Communication can only get you so far, though. There are a few other things that will help you go from exhausted parents to adventurous lovers again:

- *Lock it up and put a bell on it.* While it's not an issue when you're dealing with infants, it won't be long before your toddler is into everything—including your bedroom, your bathroom and your sex toy drawer. If your bedroom doesn't have a lock—get one. Ditto for your sex toy drawer/closet and any other space that is designated adults only. The bell is for the kid's bedroom door. If you hear it ring while you're in the middle of something naughty, you'll know there's a child headed your way.

- *Date each other.* You thought you got to stop dating because you got married, right? Nope. No one likes the idea of scheduling sex, but date nights are lifesavers for a relationship whether sex is the end result or not. You *need* the occasional dinner or movie or walk in the park alone with your spouse with your attention, your touch and your gaze focused completely on each other.

- *Get help.* Having a reliable babysitter to take care of your munchkin(s) is great for peace of mind and date nights. If money is especially tight, consider a babysitting swap or co-op with other parents so you can get in at least two date nights a month. For me, the money we pay for a Friday night sitter is worth every penny and I'd happily sacrifice something else to maintain that one-on-one time.

- *Think outside the box.* Remember making out in the backseat of the car when you were a teenager? Or sneaking a quickie in your dorm room while your roommate was in the shower? Or waking up in the middle of the night and reaching for your sleeping lover? You have to get *imaginative* once you have kids and find ways to be spontaneous. You used to find a way to have sex no matter what the obstacles. It's time to stretch those creative muscles again and get busy.

• *Nap times and bedtime are your time.* Make the most of those two-hour toddler naps on the weekend while you still have them. Sometimes you'll need a nap, too—but when you don't…find something else to do with your time. (And I'm not talking about cleaning the kitchen.) Likewise, establishing a regular bedtime for your child(ren) means you have a few built-in hours of free time at night. Of course you have a hundred things to do with those few precious hours—just make sure you add doing your partner to the list once in a while.

Repeat after me: They won't be babies (toddlers, preschoolers, et cetera) forever. Whatever stage you are dealing with, whether it's sleeping through the night or teething or terrible twos or fear of the closet monster—this too shall pass. Try to enjoy it as best you can because they won't be little for long. And during the times when you can't enjoy it, grit your teeth and bear it. Eventually, they *have* to sleep. Caffeine is your friend. So is exercise. And so is that babysitter I mentioned earlier.

Think sexy until you can be sexy. For couples whose time is at a premium and foreplay is a distant memory, keeping the lust alive is all about staying in touch with your sexual self even if it's only to text your spouse to say, *I'm going to fuck your brains out when this kid goes to kindergarten.*

SENSUAL SUGGESTIONS: PLAYTIME FOR PARENTS

Being parents is hard work, but sometimes you just have to make some time to play together. Having a playful sense of imagination can turn tired parents into desired partners once again.

1. Apply a temporary tattoo to a place hidden by your clothes. Tell your partner it's there—somewhere—and it's his job to kiss his way to its location.

2. Indulge yourselves once in a while and buy a new toy (vibrating or otherwise) that you can use during naptime, quiet time or after bedtime. Stock up on batteries and don't forget to share!

3. After the kids go to bed, play a game of strip... whatever. Monopoly, Candy Land, Hungry, Hungry Hippos—they can all be used for your own naughty pleasure. You'll never look at kids' games the same way again!

EROTIC FICTION

JUST THE TWO OF US

CHRISTOPHER COLE

My father wasn't around much when I was growing up so I was determined I was going to be there for my kids. Nobody really tells fathers how to be good fathers, though. Maybe there are serious books out there, but most of the parenting stuff I read for fathers was tongue-in-cheek with no real expectation that Dad was going to be anything but a backup parent. So when I got laid off from my job and my wife and I decided I'd be the stay-at-home parent, I wasn't sure how to do that and I flailed about for a while figuring it out. But once I had the Dad thing down (or was at least confident that I could manage three kids and make dinner at the same time without anyone getting hurt or dinner getting burned), I looked around and realized I was missing something really important: my wife.

$\mathcal{M}$ ac and cheese, hot dogs, something green," I mutter to myself, pawing through the pantry.

"Dad, I want tacos," says the four-year-old.

"Madonnacheeeeburr!" yells the two-year-old from the living room. I translate it to "McDonald's cheeseburger," something he's not even allowed to have and I didn't realize he was able to say. There go our weekly trips to the golden arches' play land and the thirty minutes of furtive writing I sometimes manage to get in on my iPhone.

The baby wails from his high chair, the most easily placated of the three. I throw some Cheerios in his direction and pull some Kraft macaroni and cheese out of the pantry.

"Sorry guys, Mommy won't be home until late so we're having hot dogs and macaroni and cheese." I start a pot of water boiling on the stove. "And green beans," I add as an afterthought, finding a package of microwavable steam-in-the-bag beans in the freezer.

I've lost them. The older two have wandered off to watch "The Wild Kratts" and the baby is chowing down on Cheerios and a cracker that presumably (hopefully) his older brother gave him. I sigh at the lack of appreciation my creative meal planning has garnered and set to making a toddler feast. It's not McDonald's, but thirty raucous minutes later, the four of us are sitting around the dinner table and they're actually consuming food instead of flinging it at each other or feeding it to the dog.

"We ate all the hot dogs," the four-year-old points out. "What's Mommy gonna eat?"

I smile. "I'll make something special for Mommy."

"Ma-ma-ma-ma," the baby coos. Figures that I'm the one home with him all day and his first word is *mama*.

An hour later, I'm tucking the boys into bed and giving them each a turn on the phone to say a quick good night to my wife. Video calls helps them—they like to kiss her image before they go to sleep—but it's hard for my wife. She doesn't usually miss bedtime, maybe two or three nights a month, but it's her favorite time because they're warm and cuddly. I prefer the mornings when they're just getting up, little wild things with enough energy to power a generator.

Bedtime for the older two is accomplished with a minimum of fuss, then I carry my phone into the baby's room to let my wife peek in on him before I tuck him in his crib. He nods sleepily as he curls up with his stuffed bear, and I hear her sigh as I turn off the light and slip out of the room.

"I'm sorry. I'll be home soon," she says, and I hear the catch in her voice as I carry my phone into our bedroom to finish the call. I can see her eyes bright with tears, the harsh fluorescent lighting in her office making her look tired and worn down.

"Hey," I tell her, smooshing my face up against the phone's camera so that she laughs. "It's okay. We're okay. They're fine and happy and healthy and you'll be here in the morning to wake them up."

Her eyes are bright with unshed tears. "I know. I just miss them... and you."

Now I'm swallowing past the lump in my throat. "Get your work done and get home, woman," I say, masking emotion with gruffness. "And I'll show you how much I miss you."

She sighs. "I wish I wasn't so tired."

I don't have an answer for that. I know she's tired. I'm tired, too. We need a vacation, but we can't afford a vacation. We need time away from the kids, but our parents live in different states, and the baby is still too young. The time will come when all three kids are in school and the job market improves so we can both work and afford vacations. But that time isn't now, and we have to suck it up.

We say our good-byes, she promises to be home in an hour and I'm left brooding on the couch. I don't have the answers for everything, but maybe, just maybe I have an answer for tonight. Maybe, just for tonight, we can forget we're broke and tired most of the time and just be us for a few hours.

By the time I hear my wife's car in the driveway, I'm feeling a little silly. I look around the love nest I've created. It's a little cool and cramped, but I think it'll work. Two candles flicker on the railing—there would be more, but I was afraid it would cause a fire. There's a battery-operated lantern as a centerpiece, a plate of antipasto foraged from the refrigerator, a loaf of crusty bread, a bowl of olive oil with herbs and a bottle of red wine that some friends brought over for a dinner party last Christmas that we never got around to opening.

I'd left a note for her so she could find me once she checks on the kids, knowing she'd never think to look here. It's close to nine o'clock and the crickets are loud, a symphony of noise that suddenly stops when my wife opens the back door and steps outside. I wait for her to pick her way across the yard, around the scattered toys, and find me.

"What in the world are you doing up there?" she asks, tired amusement in her voice.

I poke my head out of the second story of the kids' fort. "Um, surprising you?"

She's beautiful, my wife. Even after a decade, three kids and a twelve-hour workday, she's still the most beautiful woman I've ever seen. The moon kind of glints off her hair, a shade I call honey and she calls boring. It's striking in this light, falling in soft waves to her shoulders. She's still dressed for work, the ubiquitous blouse and skirt, but she's barefoot. I imagine her shoes are kicked off by the back door. There's something unbelievably sexy about this shoeless woman in work clothes.

"Come on up here," I say, extending a hand.

She laughs, sounding tired but happy. With the ease of the mother of three boys, she climbs the fort ladder and takes my hand so I can pull her up the last stretch to the platform. Her skirt hikes up to her upper thigh, and I'm not complaining one little bit.

"I've got a surprise for you."

She takes in the candles, the food and the sleeping bag tucked into the alcove behind me. "I see that. Backyard camping?" I pour her a glass of wine. "More like backyard romance. I don't think we can sleep up here."

As if to prove my point, the fort gives a bit of a creaking sigh and we both laugh, hands clamped over our mouths to prevent the sound from carrying and waking curious little boys. We've gotten used to being quiet, to whispering our conversations and occasional arguments, to muffling our moans of pleasure and giggles of delight. It is the way parents learn to maintain an adult relationship once children come along. In hushed tones and whispered sighs. Eye contact and body language. We've been doing this parenting thing long enough to know that if the kids wake up now, our fun is ruined. And neither of us wants that.

"What did you have in mind?" she asks, nibbling a Kalamata olive. "Some gymnastics on the monkey bars?"

"I hadn't thought of that. No, I was thinking some old-fashioned canoodling right here in Fort Hanky Panky."

She does her best not to roll her eyes at my 1950s slang. She doesn't succeed. "Seriously, who talks like that?"

I wrap an arm around her waist and haul her across my lap, careful of the spread I've laid out. "I talk like that," I say, channeling Clark Gable and putting a little growl in my words. "And you're my woman and you'll like it."

There's laughter, yes, but there is also her mouth against the pulse in my neck. And damn, just like that, I'm rock hard. She giggles against my throat, worrying her tongue over my pulse as she wiggles her ass on my bulge.

"Nice," she breathes against my skin, and I can't do a damned thing but nod and swallow. Somehow I think Gable would play it more suave, but who the hell cares?

We're touching each other in that familiar way of long-married couples. Her nails gently scratching the back of my neck and down between my shoulder blades; mine making circles on her bare thigh, moving steadily inward. When my fingertips grazed the lace of her panties, she gasps and I groan. How long has it been since we made out like this? It's familiar, yes, but there is also an added level of excitement. Being outside, being six feet off the ground, being out of earshot of the kids—whatever it is, it's got us both tugging at clothing and seeking the warmth of bare skin.

She tugs her panties down to midthigh while I get my pants open. There isn't a lot of room up here, and the fort creaks ominously anytime we put too much weight on one section. Best not to think about what might happen should the whole bit collapse while we're in it. The thought—us sprawled half-naked in the unmown lawn amongst the splintered wood—makes me laugh. She looks at me as if I've lost my mind.

"This is not a good time to be laughing," she says, taking my cock in her hand with a firm, no-nonsense grasp. "Not if you want to get laid."

"Yes, ma'am."

Properly chastised, I lean against the fort wall and close my eyes. A few strokes in and I've forgotten about the potential disaster we might inflict on the fort or that the neighbors might overhear my sounds of pleasure.

"Don't get too far ahead of me, mister," she mutters, hiking her skirt up and straddling my lap. "I want mine, too."

And then I'm inside her. A sensation so natural and familiar that it feels like home. She slides down on me, soft and wet. Hands braced on my shoulders, she rests her forehead against mine, her hair a silky curtain shielding us from the outside world. It's dark out here, but I stare into her eyes as she rides me, watch the way her lashes flutter as she bites her lip to keep from crying out. I arch my hips, pushing deeper into her, just to see her lose control and whimper. The crickets sing their song and we sing ours—quietly, rhythmically, our breath synchronized.

There's something to be said for being together as long as we have. Something to be celebrated in the way she knows to swivel her hips to drive me crazy and nip my neck in just the right place to make me buck into her with no thought but release. But I know her, too, and I know to slide my hands up her thighs so that my thumbs meet at her clit, massaging circles as she rides me, teasing that bit of sweet flesh that swells and aches for touch. Now we're both right there, letting go, freefalling together in a way that is a rare and special animal.

She tucks her head against my shoulder, her breath hot on my cheek. I grip her ass in my hands, pulling her closer, anchoring us together. Here beneath a star-dotted sky in a kids' fort that was never meant for this kind of fun, we are just us, her and me. Years from now, when the boys are grown, and off to college and lives of their own, this is the way it will be again. Just the two of us.

"Hey there," I say, kissing her forehead. "Welcome home."

"Hey, yourself." She sounds drowsy, relaxed. "Missed you."

"I'm right here, baby. Right here."

She nods, her hair brushing against the stubble on my cheek. "Good. I forget sometimes."

"I'll keep reminding you," I promise.

And I will.

EROTIC FICTION

THIS MOMENT

KRISTINA WRIGHT

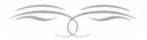

My husband and I got married in our twenties, but we didn't have children until we were in our forties. After nearly two decades as a couple with all the freedom that goes along with that, we were suddenly sharing a home with small, demanding creatures who sapped our energy and free time. I wouldn't say we felt like strangers—we'd known each other over half our lives, after all—but for a while it did feel like we were two ships passing in the night. We had to make a conscientious effort to rediscover us—the us we were before we had kids. The us that was still very much the heart of our new family.

We are so tired, we can barely find the time to talk in complete sentences.

"He's waking up," he says, shuffling into the kitchen, his hair tousled and three days' growth of beard making him look as ragged as I feel. "Bottle?"

I tilt my head toward the counter. "There."

His eyes scan the counter and skip right over the prepared bottle. "Where?"

I sigh and stand up, biting back something unkind. He's as tired as I am, I know. But why, oh why, do I always feel like the caretaker whether the baby is awake or not?

"Here," I say, picking up the bottle and putting it in his hands. "Better go before—"

As if on cue, I hear the baby wail.

"Thanks," he says, dropping a kiss on my forehead before heading upstairs to feed the baby.

It's midnight and I've just finished washing bottles and doing another load of laundry. I should crawl into bed and get a couple of hours' sleep while I can, while he has the baby and the next feeding is still two or three hours away. Instead, I sit at the kitchen table and cry.

We weren't always like this. Oh no. We were young once, we had energy, we had lives that didn't revolve around bottles and diapers and the cries of a tiny dictator. We were wrapped up in each other so well and for so long I didn't think anything could ever unravel us. But like one of those ridiculous wraps someone got me for a baby shower gift—the kind that are incredibly complicated to put on—we'd started to unravel and I couldn't figure out how to tuck the ends back around each other to keep us from falling apart. I suppose we're still young, chronologically speaking, but that tiny dictator makes us feel so very, very old. I rest my head in my hands and close my eyes.

The dream is always the same. We're on a beach, the wind is filled with the taste of salt and the sound of gulls. I'm leaning forward, elbows on my knees, staring out at the ocean, white-capped waves rolling in. Jay is sitting behind me on one of those lounge chairs, massaging sunscreen into my sun-warmed shoulders. I'm making those low pleasing sounds in my throat, the ones that sound sexual even though his hands are only stroking my shoulders.

"You need to rest," he murmurs in my ear, his tongue teasing the lobe. "You're going to crash if you don't rest."

"I am resting. Look, this is me resting."

"That's not resting. That's survival. I mean real rest."

I feel my shoulders tense. I don't want to be lectured; I want this massage. I want to rest, but I can't. I can't rest, but I can't remember why I can't rest. I have to do something. In the dream, I struggle to stand up from the chair, my legs tangling with Jay's. I start crying.

"I have to go," I cry, as he pulls me down and holds me close. "I have to go."

"Why?"

I shake my head because I can't tell him why. I don't know why. I just know I have something to do. Something that seems far more important than watching the ocean and getting my shoulders massaged with sunscreen.

"I have to go!"

I awake with a start, Jay's hands on my shoulders just as they were in the dream. I fight my way out of the sleep-induced haze, swearing I can still smell the salt of the ocean. The gulls I heard must have been the baby's cries, but all is quiet now. He's asleep. Relief, along with the desire to climb back into my dream and sleep myself, overwhelms me.

"You were having a nightmare," Jay says softly. "Where did you have to go?"

I laugh, sounding like I'm on the edge of a breakdown. "Probably to take care of the baby. We were at the beach again."

I'd told him about my dream. We don't have much time to talk anymore, and when we do it seems like it's all about baby stuff, but those few minutes over breakfast before the baby wakes up or at night before we both go to sleep for a few precious hours, we talk. We talk about what it will be like when Scottie is a little older and sleeping through the night. We talk about how wonderful it will be when we can leave him with a sitter and go out to dinner. We talk about having a normal sex life again—someday. But mostly we talk about how amazing our little boy is and how happy we are, even if we are exhausted. And he is and we are, but right now, as tired and frustrated and, yes, lonely as I am, it's hard to remember all the good.

"Come upstairs," Jay says, even before the tears start falling. "I ran a bath for you."

"You did?"

"I did."

I let him lead me up the stairs, treading carefully and quietly so that I don't wake the baby. It's amazing how sensitive I've become to noise—how quiet I am now that any disturbance might mean the difference between a two-hour nap or no nap at all. Me, who used to turn up the stereo until the windows vibrated. Now I find myself whispering even when I'm away from the baby. Which isn't often.

I smell the bath salts before he even opens the bathroom door. The only light in the room comes from a half-dozen candles lining the bathroom counter. Jay helps me off with my T-shirt and yoga pants, but this is no seduction scene. He strips me quickly and efficiently, tucking his fingers in the sides of my panties and tugging them down without so much as palming me between the legs like he usually does anytime he sees me naked. I don't know whether to be relieved or hurt, but I'm too tired to feel anything at all as he takes my hand and supports me as I lower myself into the tub. It's hot—almost too hot—just the way I like it.

I let out a breath I didn't know I'd been holding as I sink down to my chin. My eyes flutter closed, exhaustion washing over me even as the hot water relaxes the knots in my shoulders. When I open my eyes again, Jay is sitting beside the tub, smiling. He looks almost as tired as I feel. Almost. I know that we're in this together, but the physical and hormonal component of pregnancy and childbirth and postpartum takes its toll—and even now, five months later, I'm still not myself. I'm still not...me.

"What?" I ask, feeling oddly shy under his steady gaze.

It's ridiculous, of course. We've been together forever—or at least it feels like it—and he's seen me at my best and at my worst. The worst being the past six months. No, make that the past year. I have nothing to hide from him; he's seen every stretch mark and every scar, and experienced every emotion on my roller-coaster ride to motherhood. None of that matters now, as he's looking at me like he might eat me up—and I'm feeling like I might enjoy that right now.

"You're just so beautiful," he whispers.

He whispers a lot too now, my Jay. Not because he's as sensitive to noise as I am, and not because he's afraid of waking the baby. He whispers for me. Because he knows I can't handle the noise, because he empathizes with this ride I'm on even if he can't completely understand it. He whispers, he makes me hot tea and he remembers to empty the diaper pail. There are other things, bigger things, but right now, in this time and place we're at in our lives together, it's these little things that keep me sane and help me survive. It's so silly, really. I know that. But the little things are what make the difference for me. Little things like a hot bath with my favorite bath salts that smell like the ocean.

"Want to join me?"

I sound more like the exhausted mother than the seductive ingénue, but Jay doesn't seem to care. His smile widens and he suddenly doesn't look tired at all. "Sure, if you want me to."

He's so careful with me now. So thoughtful. I can feel the tears starting again, but I blink them away. "Yeah, I want you to," I say, my voice sounding husky, teasing. Maybe there is some of the ingénue left in me, after all.

He stands and strips off his T-shirt and pants, naked before I can even sit up in the bath and make room for him. He slips in behind me and I can't help but smile as I first see, then feel, his growing erection as he lowers himself into the tub and I lean back against him. Water sloshes over the edge, but there's a towel there and no need to worry about cleaning up. I can forget about the soap scum on the tile because I can't even see it in the candlelight. I don't have anything to do right this moment except enjoy a hot bath with my husband.

This brief moment of stillness and freedom instills a strange sense of exhilaration in me that masks my bone-deep exhaustion. I twist my head and stretch up to kiss him. He's not expecting it—he's expecting a quick thank-you peck, I can tell by the tenseness of his lips—but he quickly adjusts. My tongue teases the crease of his lips, and his mouth softens under mine. I feel the quick catch of his breath—or is that me?—and then we're kissing, and I'm reaching up my arm to wind it around his neck and support this odd position I'm in.

He realizes after a moment that I must be uncomfortable. "This isn't going to help your shoulders," he murmurs against my mouth, though he doesn't do anything to stop. In fact, he cups my breasts in his hands and supports their weight, just beneath the surface of the water.

I laugh. "Good point."

I stop kissing him—there will be time for that after—and rest my head in the hollow of his shoulder. My back pressed to his chest, his erection nudging me in a familiar way. How long has it been since we've had sex in the bathtub? I can't even remember. Before the baby, probably before I even got pregnant. A long time. Too long.

I lean forward, giving him room to slide farther down in the tub. It's a nice-sized bathtub and there's room for both of us to fit comfortably. So it's easy enough for me to straddle his hips and lower myself on his erection—which is exactly what I do. I know he's expecting it, even if I haven't said it, but his surprised grunt as I take him inside me makes me feel more feminine than I've felt in a very, very long time.

We've had sex since the baby—sooner than we were supposed to, actually. Here and there, in the early morning hours and late, late at night. It's good between us, always has been, but we're still in the survival part of parenting, this first year of little sleep and unpredictable schedules. It's an amazing time, so many new things to learn and watch and share, a child that is both him and me and also his own entity altogether, and I wouldn't change it for the world. But right now, in this bathtub with the now lukewarm water sloshing over the sides, this is what I need more than anything in the world.

This sense of fullness, completeness, I know it so well and yet it feels like it's been so long since I felt him. His cock pressing up into me, stretching me, filling me, making me feel whole; his teeth pressing against my neck, hands on my hips, then my breasts, then tugging at my hair. Rocking into me slowly, hitting that sweet spot that makes me so much wetter, slicker in a way that water doesn't. I whimper, softly, always softly, but it echoes off the bathroom tile. The noise doesn't bother me though. I need this; I need the physical release and the vocal release. I whimper again as he pushes into me and then glides back, making a wave that splashes up my chest.

He's whispering in my ear, nonsensical things that would make me laugh in other circumstances. "Beautiful girl, so pretty, so wet and slippery, my mermaid girl," a silly, sexy love song from my beloved.

I grip the edge of the tub to give him some resistance, tightening my muscles inside to hold him, relaxing so that my pussy ripples along the length of him. His words fade away and become soft moans, softer than mine, quiet and intense, focused at the point where he is so far inside me it almost hurts. I rock against him, trying to coax those moans out of him.

"Louder," I whisper so softly I know he probably doesn't hear me.

But he does, and when I twist my hips just so, he groans in that way that lets me know he's close. I am right there on the edge of orgasm and I thrust back against him hard, feeling muscles I haven't used in a long time straining in unison toward that release. And then I'm there, and he is too, judging by the way he's grinding against me, his cock feeling thicker, harder inside me. We're there, together, coming and gasping and groaning. Over the edge like water over the lip of the bathtub, falling, falling...

The water feels almost cold by the time my breathing returns to normal and my thigh muscles stop quivering. I'm lying against him, relaxed, limp, half-asleep. All of the hard edges of the day have been softened; everything is a sweet, languid blur.

"We should probably get up," Jay says, though he doesn't move. "You need to get some sleep."

"I'm fine," I tell him. And I am. "I don't care about sleep. Not right now."

And it's true—I don't care. We get so few of these moments together now—stolen fragments of time scattered across a canvas of busy days and tired nights. Days and weeks and months blending and blurring as we find our center through this new life. It's a beautiful, amazing life and every moment—including *this* moment—is precious.

FIVE

MIDDLE-AGED LUST...
AND BEYOND—GROW OLD
ALONG WITH ME

Only people in their twenties are having good sex. That's the message I get everywhere I look, from magazines to movies. Even the self-help books at the bookstore have some young twentysomething chick on the cover, telling me my sex life would be better if only I looked like her. But there must be a lot of people old enough to be grandparents and members of AARP who have fantastic sex lives, right? I wish I heard more about those people.

—Renee, married twenty-seven years

*I*n a youth-obsessed culture, it can seem like the only people having sex are a decade (or two, or three) younger than you. We're inundated with youthful images of love and sex. Every Hollywood love story seems to be about two college kids falling in love. (And one of them may or may not be a vampire, werewolf or superhero.) The explosion of young-adult literature coupled with youthful protagonists in the blockbuster *Fifty Shades of Grey* trilogy make it seem as if the whole world is younger, richer, more interesting and better looking. (Please tell me it's not just me who feels this way.)

It's easy to see why committed couples get discouraged when they hit a dry patch in their sex lives. Even the self-help books and magazine articles seem to be talking to a younger readership. A single readership. A readership that knows nothing about decades of sharing parenting and household responsibilities and the need to carve out couple-time amid cleaning out the garage and planning the family reunion. But we're out here, millions of us, fighting the good fight and maintaining happy, *sexy* relationships in the long term. We are just doing it quietly because the youth-centered media is more interested in covering the latest teen crush sensation than interviewing average people in average places who happen to be having rocking sex behind closed doors.

There was a collective "ewww" from the youth-centered media a couple of years ago when Jane Fonda was quoted as saying, "At seventy-four, I have never had such a fulfilling sex life. When I was young I had so many inhibitions—I didn't know what I desired." Meanwhile, the over-forty crowd was smiling and nodding and thinking, "Yeah, I'm looking forward to that," because they know there's no expiration date for a satisfying sex life. There can be a number of factors impacting a couple's sex life, but there is no magic age when good sex dries up and disappears. Use it or lose it, as the old adage goes, and there is increasing evidence that the physical and mental benefits of sex continue well into old age.

As Dr. Gail Saltz explains in her 2009 book *The Ripple Effect: How Better Sex Can Lead to a Better Life*, "Unlike in Vegas, what happens in bed doesn't stay in bed. It emanates outward in every direction, until it reaches the farthest shores of family, friendships, and work." Instinctively, we all know this. Good sex makes us happy. Good sex gets us through the bad stuff. Good sex helps us connect even when we're arguing about private school versus public school or crossover SUV versus hybrid sedan. Good sex fulfills our need to connect with our spouse, but it can also be a balm for frustrations and disappointments—not to mention a terrific sleep aid when you're stressed. Study after study shows the benefits of sex range from improving your mood to toning your muscles, but really, the main reason to carve out some precious time for each other is simple: you're in this for the long haul and it's important to maintain the most intimate aspect of your relationship.

I don't know too many people who are still bragging about their sex lives ten, fifteen, twenty years into their marriage. For one, we've (mostly) matured and no longer feel the need to rate and compare ourselves next to our friends. For another, there is some cultural gag order that's issued on married people who have made it past the first few years of marriage and are still having good sex. We're not *supposed* to talk about it once we've passed the seven year itch or had a couple of kids or have more gray hair than not. It's almost taboo. We are supposed to complain that we haven't had sex since Clinton was in office and that once you have kids sex is a thing of the past. I've been in more than one group conversation that went something like this:

Woman A: We used to have sex three times a day. Then we had kids and got old.

Woman B: Three times a day? We maybe had it three times a week. Now it's three times a year.

Woman C: I'm too tired for sex. I'm too tired to even think about sex.

Woman A: I miss sex, but there's no time. Kids, work, life. You know what I mean. I feel like I have to schedule sex and who wants to do that?

Woman B: Sex is overrated anyway.

Woman C: Sex is for teenagers.

Woman A: God, my kids are almost teenagers. They're going to be having more sex than me soon. Of course, any sex would be more sex than me.

And so it goes. Men complain about not having sex, too. As if the man who has gone the longest without having sex is entitled to some kind of an award. But there is no award for *not* having sex. Sex is its own reward. We used to know this instinctively. It's the reason we were willing to drive all night to visit a girlfriend at college or shave our legs in the dead of winter just in case there was a chance of getting lucky with the cute guy at work. Sex is *sublime.* We get wrapped up in the minutiae of life and forget and need to be reminded of that. But if both partners forget the veritable banquet of treats of a good sex life, what's left? Two people who vaguely remember having good sex?

You might hit a patch in middle age where you honestly don't think you'll ever want to have sex again. You may feel the need to mourn your younger sexual self or you might not even miss it. But things change—people change—and your sex drive also changes, for a variety of reasons. It's important to understand that there are a number of factors involved in having a good sex life and that the physical and mental changes of aging can play a huge role in how you feel about sex and in how much you enjoy sex. It's important to not only talk to your partner about your needs and what you want for yourself as part of a couple, but to also talk to your doctor about any changes that may be affecting your sexual interest or pleasure. Don't assume that just because you've hit forty, fifty or beyond, you're not supposed to still want and enjoy sex. Age is just a number—and good sex can be yours for the taking regardless of age.

Donna George Storey's "Vintage Love" recounts a marriage filled with intimate, erotic encounters that have only improved with the years. This is the story your long-married friends don't tell—or maybe it's the story *you* don't tell your younger friends for fear it makes you seem...scandalously improper. To hell with our youth-obsessed culture, we of the silver strands and crow's feet need to shout our sexual satisfaction from the rooftops and beyond. We need to represent, as the younger generation might say. The sex may involve fewer bendy positions (or maybe not—those Pilates and yoga classes come in handy, don't they?) and may not match the Hollywood twenty-something versions of sex, but it's *your* sex and, damn, it should be everything you want it to be. Sure, life is going to throw us curveballs like menopause, as Robin Elizabeth Sampson writes about in "Doing It All Wrong," but that's life. Try a different swing (or a little lube) and hit it out of the park.

Whether your sex life is thirty amazing years and going strong or in need of a little work, or still in the early stages and seems like it'll never wane—make a vow not to forget about sex. Promise each other that you will remember that sex is good and that good sex can not only be orgasmic, but also therapeutic. Don't forget the benefits of sex are emotional and physical. It not only feels good, it makes you feel younger, healthier and more confident. I'm not saying do it no matter what—I'm saying no matter what, make some time for each other and see where it takes you.

SENSUAL SUGGESTIONS: AGING WITH GRACE

The benefits of growing older include confidence in who you are. Be your best self with the person who loves you most.

1. Play hooky from work and meet each other for a matinee movie. See how far you're willing to go in a dark, empty theater even after all these years.

2. It can be fun—and sexy—to share a new passion with your partner.

Find something you're both interested in—playing the guitar, learning a language, taking up hiking— anything that gets you out of the house and doing something new together.

3. Renew your vows. It can be as simple as a back- yard BBQ or as fancy as a beachfront extravaganza. A renewal of your vows is a recommitment to each other—and a chance to take another (or first!) honey- moon.

EROTIC FICTION

VINTAGE LOVE

DONNA GEORGE STOREY

As much as I like to think I'm immune to media images, I know they've shaped my imagination, especially when it comes to sexual desire. Sexy people are always young and perfectly toned. Their pleasure is easily quantifiable in the dozens of hot lovers they collect, the hours he can stay hard, the impressive tally of her multiple orgasms. Sex for anyone over forty is visible only in Viagra commercials where a silver-haired couple shows off their dentures on the beach at sunset. Skeptical as I was of media lies, I still assumed that the quality of my sex life would decline with age. Yet, as my husband and I grew older together, we discovered the true meaning of eroticism: the feelings, memories, intimacy and trust that transform a physical act into a rich communion. How happy I am that the ad men got that wrong, too!

I know I'm not supposed to want it anymore. I'm definitely not supposed to enjoy it as much as I do. I'm a fifty-year-old married woman. They tell me I'm invisible, which means my own sexual desire must no longer exist. If only they knew.

You're a rebel, too. Married men in their fifties are supposed to pine for women half their age. But you're still happy with what you have. You watch me undress with glowing eyes and breathe "Wow," with a passion that makes my whole body blush. Hours after we make love, you slip your arms around me and whisper, "That was amazing. When can we do it again?"

I may be well beyond my expiration date, but I, too, am allowed an occasional sexual fantasy about a young hunk with bulging biceps and washboard abs (no faces or IQs required) or a suave billionaire who sweeps me off my feet and guesses my every depraved desire without a word spoken. But I'd rather get tingly imagining my next assignation with a slim, white-haired man I've known for twenty-seven years. How perverse I am to reject a perfect stranger for a familiar partner who has earned my trust over more than a thousand nights of pleasure.

I want to find a new word for our illicit pleasure, one that captures all of its intoxicating complexity.

Remember when we splurged on our first bottle of fine wine? It was a 1970 Château Mouton Rothschild, twenty-two years old the night we took it to a restaurant to celebrate our fifth wedding anniversary. The waiter smirked when we said we'd brought our own wine, but his eyes widened with respect when he saw the label. He whisked away the bottle—"Do you think he's coming back?" I whispered to you across the table—and returned with a crystal carafe and the open bottle, which he decanted before us. Neither of us was sure what to expect when we took the first sip, but I saw my own awe reflected in your face. I'd never tasted anything so alive, mysterious red fruits and berries I couldn't name spiked with faint echoes of oaken casks in a château cellar. I swallowed the magic liquid reluctantly, already mourning my loss, but then the oddest thing happened. A second burst of flavor exploded on my palate, this time the essence of black-currants mixed with ancient spices. I waited, my senses on high alert. The finish lingered on and on, seducing my tongue with an ever-changing dance of flavors, as if each of those twenty-two years were distilled into a unique essence.

Sex with you is like that wine.

So let's call it vintage love.

When I touch your soft skin; when I wrap my hand around your thick, sturdy cock; when I take you inside me and rub myself against your belly with total abandon, I feel the rich history of our pleasure in our flesh.

We may be erotic renegades now, but at the beginning we were straight from central casting: hot-blooded, sex-crazed twentysome-things, barely managing to stumble out of bed to refuel with food before we went at it again. Our thoughts were as intertwined as our bodies. You whispered once, as we floated in the afterglow, that you missed me before you met me. I thought that was the perfect way to express it.

I won't be a revisionist, though. We both brought issues along with us. Yours was the discrepancy in our past experience—your three lovers to my eighteen. Mine was a vow never again to mislead anyone about my orgasm or lack thereof. (I hadn't "faked it" *When Harry Met Sally*-style, but I never spoke up if a man assumed what worked for him worked for me.) Most of the time you said you enjoyed making me come, even if it "took a long time." But occasionally you'd ask peevishly if I'd be willing to comp you one. Tempted as I was to please my man, I forced myself to insist on something in return, if only your hands caressing my breasts while I played with myself. At the time, I sometimes worried you'd leave me for the perfect woman who could come in five minutes flat every time, but I wonder if I'd love sex so much today if I couldn't trust it would be equal. You grimace and say, "Boy, what an asshole I was back then," but age has brought a natural equality. Now, we're a perfect match. I love to hold you in my arms as you enjoy a leisurely finish, your ecstasy pulsing through my boneless, satisfied body.

That wasn't the only challenge we faced in the early days, was it? When I lived in Japan for that cruel, lonely year, we both wilted. Anxious to prove yourself professionally, it was hard for you to resist the pressures of your job at a start-up, with its eighty-hour workweeks and long business trips overseas.

In our early thirties we had our first child. It was joyous and exhausting to care for this helpless, adorable little human being. We didn't have intercourse for a year. It wasn't for lack of interest. Those not-so-wise experts claimed a couple could go back to having sex six weeks after the birth. When we tried, it felt like I was being jabbed with a red-hot poker. We did manage a few creative compensations, sweet oases in the desert. One night when Grandma was visiting, we rented a private room at the hot tub spa. It felt like we were having an affair. I gave you a blow job as you sat at the edge of the redwood tub, the star-filled sky arching above us. Then you strummed me to orgasm under the pulsing water. I got better at blow jobs, and we both got off when you came on my breasts. We finally made love comfortably again a few weeks before our son's first birthday. I felt as tight as a virgin and afterward cried with relief.

But that was the turning point, wasn't it? After ten years together, maybe we had been taking sex for granted. Now we treasured our erotic life, knowing it had to be nurtured, just like a child. Weekend nap times were our most reliable times to "slip it in." If the baby refused to sleep, we were all fussy for the rest of the day. When it was our turn for a night out in the babysitting share, we lied to our friends that we were going out to dinner, then rushed home to bed where we'd try out something new and moan and groan as loud as we could.

I think we have that dry year to thank for my erotica writing, too. When I left teaching, I started writing fiction during the baby's naps. Every story I wrote quickly turned to sex. Who would have thought my novice efforts would bring so much sizzle to our own bed? In my hunger to capture the truth and mystery of sex in words, I gazed and tasted and sniffed and listened more intensely than ever before. I remember running my hand over the curves of your shoulder and arm, slowly, savoring every sensation. Soon an electric warmth began to prickle in my palm and descend, gradually, to my pussy. I'd never really understood why just touching my body could turn you on so much, but I suddenly felt in my own flesh what a turn-on it could be to appreciate you so intimately. I became more daring, buying velvet gloves at the Halloween store, using a scarf to blindfold you. I'd always thought of myself as a sexual person, but I realized then that I'd let you lead the way, afraid you'd be threatened by my erotic curiosity.

We were growing up, weren't we? We both had more confidence to take risks with each other. When that female-friendly erotic store opened in town, it gave me cover to buy a few toys, rent a few videos. We still have the sensual mitten where one side is leather and the other black fur. You love it when I caress you all over with the furry side as you lie still, accepting the pleasure I give you with soft moans. I prefer a gentle spanking with the leather, one of the surprisingly erotic legacies of a Catholic upbringing where indulgence must always be tempered with penance. We also tried acting out our fantasies, very literally at first. When you told me about your Avon Lady scenario, I actually went out on the front porch with a small suitcase and rang the doorbell. Neither of us could keep a straight face when you answered the door. We decided on a very successful compromise: lying in bed naked and whispering suggestive dialogue without the awkwardness of a fully staged performance:

Did you masturbate while I was away on the business trip?

Uh, well…yeah.

What a naughty girl. You know there are consequences for this behavior.

I'm s-sorry. I'll try not to do it again.

Good intentions for the future hardly matter now. Tell me what a proper punishment is for a wife who masturbates when her husband is away.

Ah, um, a spanking on my naughty behind?

Exactly. Turn over on your stomach.

You always played it perfectly. You didn't judge or ridicule. As I wrote more stories, we researched things we'd never tried before. That's how we had anal intercourse for the first time. Of course we read a book first. We always read books before we try something adult and intimidating like buying a house or hiring a contractor. Backdoor sex required care, but it wasn't as painful as I feared. Instead it gave us both a soaring sense of victory, as if we were graduating to a more advanced level of sophistication in bed. Yet once we earned our anal sex badge, we came to prefer the gentler and more mutual forms of anal eroticism. Fingers gently circling rings of muscle, tiny drumlike taps on the tender opening, a fingertip inserted during orgasm. They say every couple thinks they discovered sex, but over the years we truly did discover our own rhythm and style.

Midlife brought more challenges. Career changes and a parent's death. Our bodies have changed, although in some ways we're healthier and more mindful. There's no question that we both bear scars of life's wounds, some more visible than others, even pain we inflicted on each other. Yet surviving those hard times together and moving on to a healing place only deepened our trust in the end. We've proven we will not abandon each other once it isn't fun and easy anymore. After all, the best grapes develop their character in stony soil.

Now we joke that we have to do it as often as possible because we don't know what the future will bring. You'd never see this in a movie, but vintage sex is better than ever. I've never felt as supremely contented as I do after we make love. Let's be honest, we're both more cheerful for days afterward. A roll in the sheets takes the edges off of life's annoyances, makes us kinder and reminds us of the most special, private connection we have. When I was younger I used to roll my eyes at those earnest types who prettified a sweaty, carnal deed by calling it "sacred." At fifty, I finally understand what they mean.

As for buying the story that middle-aged soccer parents have the best years of their sex lives well behind them? Well, just tell me which days you're working from home next week. I'm blocking out those lunch hours in my planner.

I can picture now exactly how it will be. I'll get ready a little early so I can leave the day's distractions outside the bedroom door. I'll undress, lay out our "fuck towel." Slipping under the blankets to warm the bed, I'll close my eyes and focus on the quickening of excitement in my belly. I know it's going to be good. Because you know just how to transport me to that magical place where mind and body float in timeless pleasure. You'll kiss and tweak my nipples lightly, then harder as my skin flushes and sweats. You'll slip your finger in the groove just to the right of my clitoris and strum until the diamond swells. You'll know to hold still when I'm on top, so that I can thrust against your belly and get the right friction. Maybe we'll add in something a little edgy. We'll whisper a fantasy about you fucking my ass in your office, or we'll get out the feather duster and I'll brush you all over, and then you'll tease my clit with the end of the handle. I'll take charge and wrap my lips around the purple helmet of your cock and tap your sensitive back hole until you moan. Or maybe we'll just make love in silence, missionary-style, no special tricks, as if we were repressed Victorians. That sly form of psychological bondage is a surprising turn-on to us both.

But I forget myself. We're not supposed to do these things at our age. Which might be part of the reason we're having such a wonderful time.

Like that first-growth Bordeaux of twenty years past, our vintage love reveals its finest pleasures only to those patient enough to wait, savor and enjoy.

Thank you for every delicious day—and night—of our journey together.

EROTIC FICTION

DOING IT ALL WRONG

ROBIN ELIZABETH SAMPSON

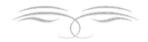

My husband and I have been married for more than thirty years. We've raised three children and are now preparing to move to another state and get on with the next stage of our lives. I've been thinking a lot about how come we still enjoy sex with each other so much, when so often it's assumed that couples together as long as we've been are past that. I don't honestly know.

*I*t's just past four in the morning and I can't get back to sleep. The rearranged room is unfamiliar enough that I had to fully wake up to make my way to the bathroom in the dark. Back under the covers, I check my cell phone that now doubles as an alarm clock in this "home-staged" bedroom. Four sixteen A.M. I sense my husband stir next to me, but don't ask, "Are you awake?"

Exhausted the night before, after a day of driving in rain only to come home to sad news, I'd read only about two pages of a memoir before I gave in and turned out the light. Half-asleep by the time my husband came to bed, I was somewhat sad that he didn't cuddle up to me. It had been more than a week since the last time we'd had sex. With so much for us both to do, we'd just been too tired each night. Last night was no different. I soon was asleep.

My dreams these days reflect my anxieties about our planned move. The kids are grown, for the most part moved out, so my husband and I are going to pursue our dream of building a cabin in the woods. But after days spent moving furniture from room to room in order to refinish floors, or painting all the walls neutral colors, my dreams are of parking a bed in a lot, just like a car, or of being dipped in ultra-white semigloss latex paint. Nothing sexy or kinky about either of these dreams. I rarely have sex dreams anymore. At least I'm not having nightmares.

In the dark, in this pretty-much-bare room, so echoey that I removed the clock because its ticking was so annoying, I can tell from his breathing he is awake too. I reach my foot back and touch his leg, my way of letting him know I know he's awake. He turns toward me and wraps his arm around me, his hand resting on my belly. In my head, I run through a do-I-or-do-I-not-want-sex list. Not that he's yet indicated an interest. It had been a tough day, with me upset about many things, and he could just be comforting me.

I'm missing my grown daughters (one is married and lives three thousand miles away and the other is getting ready to move to the other side of the world), and I feel great sadness for a friend who just lost her mother to cancer. That makes three women friends who have lost their mothers in the past nine months. More will come, since we are of that age when we lose our parents. Yes, I'm feeling my age more and more these days. In an effort to derail this sad train of thought, I pay attention to the slight movements of my husband's fingers. I think I want sex.

I used to always want sex. Miss One-Track-Mind. That was me. Turned on at the drop of a hat or flick of a nipple. No longer. Thank you menopause. And all the more noticeable after the hyper-libido that seemed to occur in the years leading up. At times I've felt short-changed because I'd worked to get past various inhibitions and now...

Now, as I sense the tentative intention in his fingertips, I'm glad that I'm stubborn and have refused to roll over and play dead, sexually speaking. I'm glad I'm a voracious reader and came across wise words that explained that while, yes, my body's responses have changed, that is all. They've changed. Time to learn them anew. Time to have patience. Something I'm not known for. So, while I used to give up when I didn't feel that tingle at first touch, I now know that good things come to those who keep at it. Besides, I've never been a sprinter.

His hand travels a little lower, toward the crease of hip and thigh, where the hem of my T-shirt falls. While we usually sleep in the nude, last night when I got into bed to read, it was a bit chilly, so I wore an old T-shirt and then fell asleep in it. I've never been much for lingerie, being more of the old-hippy, earth-mother, nature-girl type. I mean, we still sleep in a waterbed. With an Indian-print bedspread. Yup, we're throwbacks. But that doesn't mean that I don't sometimes long for a change of pace. It's just that we're both creatures of habit. I almost hold my breath in anticipation as I feel his touch through the cloth getting closer to where there is just skin.

As his fingers brush the top of my thigh, I pay attention to my body's response, which is somewhat like a raised eyebrow—*Hmmm, what is this? I think I like this.* Arousal no longer comes with an electric shock and a flood of wetness. It is more a slow-rising tide as he draws his fingers up over my hip, raising my T-shirt ahead of them. I communicate my desire with an indrawn breath.

Our lovemaking almost always starts quietly. It's been that way from the beginning. A previous lover of mine had been prone to running commentary, and I enjoyed the quiet of the man that I would marry. But years later, wanting, needing something different, something more, some sound from him, I'd wondered why he was so quiet, and he told me that it was because it was the sounds I made, those little sounds, that turned him on. But I need his sounds too. I'm not sure we've ever gotten the whole "good communication skills" thing right. At least, I sure feel that way sometimes. By some accounts we're doing it all wrong. I should have learned by now not to read relationship advice articles, because according to them we're a disaster waiting to happen. It's been thirty-plus years. Any day now.

His hand is exploring well-traveled territory. Sometimes my mind wanders, and I've found I need to stay focused in order for the arousal to not slip away. In a way, these distractions–I forgot to call, I need to return that, I wonder how so-and-so is doing?–are like children knocking on the bedroom just as Mom and Dad start getting friendly. Somehow we managed to navigate through those years and maintain our passion for each other. I steer my attention back to his fingers, which are now reaching for a nipple. He gives it a quick tweak and I suck in breath. As I do, I can feel his cock begin to harden against the small of my back.

He plays with my breasts for a bit, and I think about how he's had to relearn my preferences for touch—ranging from gentle to rough—often over the years. Lately I've found that too much or too rough is irritating. I don't want to say "Don't do that," because I don't necessarily want him to stop, so I usually just gently touch his hand as a way of letting him know to ease up. It's not like I even know whether something will feel good or feel bothersome to me. This is new to me too. I am just happy my body is responding.

His is too. I slide my hand down behind me and grasp his growing erection. Now it is his turn to make the sounds that help turn me on.

I feel his hand move down and he starts running his knuckles up and down the cleft of my ass. I press back against him, then, frustrated with the T-shirt that is now in the way, I half sit up and remove it, almost falling over. I laugh and snuggle back against him, and he makes a contented "Mmm," as he curls around me. He reaches around and brushes against my pubic hair, then his fingers slowly find their way to my slit. As his fingers sink into me, I hear him say a muffled, "Ohh," which I know is the result of him finding me wet.

Naturally wet.

Lately, if I'm at all anticipating sex, I'll apply a little bit of lube even before getting into bed. Not because I always need it, but it seems the slickness actually makes me feel even more aroused. I've never been afraid to use lube. I want the sex to be comfortable, to feel good, so I've never been afraid to reach for the tube or bottle. I've always thought a big ol' pump bottle would be nice. Maybe when we get moved. There goes my mind wandering again, though at least it's staying in the right neighborhood, thinking about sex.

He's now stroking me, pressing and caressing, making it harder for me to be distracted. I roll onto my stomach, spread my legs so he can more easily plunge his fingers into me. I feel him slide his other arm under my stomach and reach for my clit. I gasp and find myself entering that delightful place of almost too much, but not quite. Every now and then, he'll press my clit with his fingernails, not too hard, but enough to make me moan and raise my hips off the bed. I'm not trying to get away from his touch, but I am. Getting near the edge, then pulling back, then edging forward again. It is that borderline I crave. And he knows it.

At least I think he knows it. I don't know if it's instinctual or intellectual, but he usually reads me well. And I hope I read him well. At least we both know that we can't always get it right. But usually we do. He knows that I need much more manual stimulation these days.

His fingers work me into a frenzy, and when he reaches to shift us so he can enter me, I quickly reach down and touch my cunt, testing for dryness, since I know that if I'm not wet enough when he tries to enter me, I won't like it. Some friction is good. Too much is just asking for trouble. I reach into the drawer beneath the bed for the lube.

My fingers gently apply enough to ease the way. I am wanting him inside me. When he hears the click of the lid closing, I hear his breathing quicken. He lifts my leg and I position him and he pushes and gasps and I am filled and it doesn't matter how many times I've felt this, I love it. I love the feel of him entering me. Then we begin to fuck. We press and rub together. Slowly. Faster. We twist our bodies, pause, readjust covers, grip hips, hold, plunge, rest and fuck and fuck and fuck. We lose ourselves. We stop thinking about what we are doing and just do.

This is what we do right. We both know how to let go. Not that we always do, but most of the time, we let our animal bodies take over and take us to that place where there are no boxes to pack, or walls to paint, or floors to refinish, or bills to worry about, or car troubles, or next year's tuition, or that sensitive tooth or...

There is only skin and breath. Heartbeats and hands. The everyday transcendent. At that moment, just before climax, we are stronger, we are younger, we are closer to each other, than at any other moment. It is for this moment that we struggle through all the others.

I can feel my orgasm teasing me. Almost. Almost. Almost. And then it is there. It is not sharp and strong, a thunderclap, like it used to be. There is subtleness, roundness to it, like rolling thunder that just keeps rumbling. And as I tremble with the aftershocks, for that is what they feel like, he pumps with a franticness, and I grip his ass with my fingers and almost will him to come. And he does, pressing into me and holding still, grasping me, breathing hard.

With a shudder and a laugh, we pull away from each other, try to find pillows and the now messed-up covers. We still have some time to sleep, and we sort of snuggle, then flop over and drift off for a couple of hours. In the morning I'll try to capture these moments with totally inadequate words.

SIX

LUST FOR BETTER OR WORSE— WHEN THE GOING GETS TOUGH

It's easy when you're young. Just starting out, broke, living paycheck to paycheck, it seems like hell—but those are the best days. When you only have each other. Now the economy is eating up our savings, the kids' needs always come first (and there is no second), I'm stressed about being downsized out of a job, my partner is talking about going back to school. We never see each other. I know it could be worse. I really do know we are lucky to still be together after all of the ups and downs. But when is it our time again?

—David, married for twelve years

$\mathcal{M}$arriage is a mystery. People can tell you what it'll be like and give you advice on how to have a happy marriage, but no two couples experience marriage the same way. Going in, you may think it's going to be wall-to-wall sex punctuated by pizza deliveries and 2:00 A.M. kitchen rendezvous to devour anything that isn't nailed down. Okay, maybe most of us don't think that (though I really do remember feeling like that for at least a few months), but most people who decide to promise "until death us do part," or some other somber equivalent, are not thinking about the long haul and the tough times when they're giddy with joy over how much sex they're going to be having for the foreseeable future. But those tough times *do* come, no matter how charmed a life you lead—and sexual intimacy is often the first casualty when life gets tough.

There are dark days in every marriage, highs and lows in every stage of commitment. The divorce statistics tell us that a lot of couples decide to go their separate ways rather than hold on through the tough times. Most marriages that end go out with a whimper instead of a bang—no pun intended. It's rarely one big cataclysmic event that ends the relationship; rather, it's the distancing that occurs over months or years. Job stress, health issues, the demands of parenting and family obligations—we all get wrapped up in the day-to-day struggles and forget about our partners. Sex slips farther and farther down the priority list, behind getting the dryer fixed and polishing the resume in case the economy dips even farther and taking the twins to ballet class, until sex—and the marriage itself—is dead last on an impossibly long to-do list for both people.

Certainly, there are legitimate reasons why couples split up—but I'm willing to bet there are a lot of good reasons to stay together, if only couples could remind themselves why they got married in the first place. Sex isn't the answer in every difficult or busy time a couple faces, but as the stories below illustrate, sex can often bridge the gaps that couples in long-term commitments often encounter. Anya Richards's "Made to Last" shows that you *can* survive the year from Hell without killing each other and do it in a way that feels like a sexual renewing of your vows. Christine d'Abo's "Now Playing" is a playful story about a clever couple stealing time from the kids, dogs and family chores in any way they can. And the truth is, that's what we have to do if we're going to make it through the times of stress and disconnection that come when real life starts knocking on—and down—the front door: steal time.

When every instinct in you is screaming to turn inward, to wrap your fear or stress or anger around you like a bulletproof blanket and protect yourself from the world, fight that urge. Reach out a hand to that person you chose as your partner and walk the road together. Whatever you're dealing with, whether it's an unpredictable financial crisis or coping with difficult family issues, you're in it together. Love has gotten you this far, and intimacy—true intimacy, not just "doing it to get it over with"—will ease some of the stress and tension. The problems you're facing will still be there in the morning, but you'll have reinforced your already strong foundation and will have a better outlook and sense of balance. (And here you thought sex was all about having an orgasm!)

Study after study indicates that stress and exhaustion wreak havoc on a couple's sex life. But sex can alleviate stress (at least temporarily) and help you relax—which means more/better sleep. So why aren't we all having sex more often? According to the National Marriage Project, couples who routinely have "couple time" are three and a half times more likely to be happy in their marriages—probably because date night often makes couples feel closer to one another—which often leads to more frequent and more satisfying sex. It's a very happy, sexy domino effect of spending quality time together regardless of what else is going on in your lives (and sometimes *because* of what else is going on) and reaping the benefits of that quality time, emotionally and sexually.

Happily married couples are not a rare statistic, despite what the media and entertainment communities would have us believe. Married couples who are sexually and emotionally satisfied are invisible in society, leading us to believe that sex beyond the honeymoon stage of life is nonexistent—and that that's okay. It's neither. In a February 2012 article for *USA Today* sex therapist and clinical psychologist Barry McCarthy, points out that society ignores marital sex. "You never see marital sex in the movies," he says. "In the movies and in our culture, what is exciting sexually is something that is breaking the boundaries and is illicit. The key to marital sex is integrating intimacy and eroticism."

But how do we do that? How do we take the intimacy that is inherent to sharing a life and keep it sexy when life is hurtling fireballs at us while we juggle a dozen different stressors? With imagination, determination and a good sense of humor, judging by the stories that have been contributed to this book. It *is* possible to have a good, satisfying sex life at every stage of your marriage even when the rest of the world seems to be going to hell and trying to take you with it. Don't let the movies, your friends or your own self-doubt tell you otherwise.

SENSUAL SUGGESTIONS:
STUCK LIKE GLUE

When life throws you a curveball, remember who is on your team. Reach out to each other when you're feeling lousy and your connection will be stronger for it.

1. Making love is not only good for your physical and mental health, it's good for your relationship. Sex can take your mind off your troubles when nothing else can.

2. If the present is weighing you down, escape to the past. Relive your best memories—go to "your" place, flirt with each other like you did back then, tap into that person you were when you could barely keep your hands off each other.

3. Talk about the future. Thinking about the good things to come will not only get your creative juices flowing—it'll make you hot for each other in a fresh new way.

EROTIC FICTION

MADE TO LAST

ANYA RICHARDS

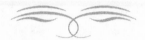

The year from Hell stretched to two, and everything that could go wrong did. For my husband and me sex wasn't the answer, but it sure went a long way toward helping us reconnect, remember what's important and release some of the pent-up stress. With a reaffirmation of the bonds we share, we were once more ready to face the world, together.

It's one o'clock in the morning, and I'm wide-awake.

This isn't anything new, unfortunately. Recently sleep has become an elusive, craved and yet frightening concept. It sometimes provides relief, sometimes makes things worse, as problems follow me into dreamland and continue their unrelenting torture.

Beside me, my husband sighs and rolls onto his side. From the tenor of his breathing I know he's dead to the world, and annoyance flashes through me. How can he sleep so soundly, night after night, while I lie awake, my brain unable to shut down long enough for me to nod off?

But I know I'm not alone with my fears. All the signs of stress are there in him too. Just this evening I looked across the living room and caught him staring out the window, eyes unfocused, fingers tapping a sharp, staccato rhythm on the arm of his chair. He's usually calm, almost serene, just the type of man a high-voltage woman like me needs. He's my anchor, the voice of reason when I'm tempted to go off the deep end. It hurts to see him obviously restless, with worry etching new lines into his beloved, beautiful face.

Staring up into the darkness, I start cataloging our problems, the relentless cycle starting anew. Instantly the muscles in my neck tighten and my stomach knots. I try to think of something else— concentrate on the plot of my latest book—but within minutes I've somehow circled back to reality. Sometimes I think I'd feel better if I could just cry, let it out, but that's not my way. Tears have always been something to avoid, repress, fight. They're a weakness I can't allow myself. If I start I might not be able to stop, and that thought scares me more than any other. For me, that heralds the onset of madness.

As though sensing my terror, my husband moves closer, his arm settling across my stomach. That simple touch, the sensation of his warmth so close, brings a sob close to the surface and I'm forced to swallow it down. I don't feel as though I deserve his affection right now. I have a sneaky suspicion the blame for our current problems rests squarely on my shoulders. Yet, it feels so good having him beside me. Instead of moving away I roll onto my side, facing away from him, and spoon closer.

"You okay, honey?"

His breath stirs my hair, and his arm tightens around me. He knows the answer to the question as well as I do but, even so, my first instinct is to reassure.

"Uh-huh. I'm fine."

His chest expands, and when he exhales it's with a quiet, disbelieving huff.

"Liar." With gentle insistence he rolls me over to face him. "I can smell the smoke from here. You can't solve anything at this time of the morning. Let it go. Get some sleep."

"Easier said than done." I loop my arms around his neck and snuggle in. "Sorry to wake you."

"It's okay." He pulls my leg up over his hip, then seems to change his mind and eases it back down a bit. "This is even better than sleep."

I don't answer, just lean against his chest and listen to his heartbeat. The problem with—and joy of—being married so long, loving someone so much, is how familiar they become. That one little movement, the shifting of my leg, tells me he's getting aroused.

We long ago discovered the major difference in how we handle stress. He wants sex all the time; needs the release of a good, hard orgasm. Me? I can hardly stand the thought of it, feeling as though what little energy I have left would be better spent getting through the day. It took some doing, but we've learned to compromise. He lets me take the lead, waiting until I initiate intimacy rather than trying to get me in the mood.

Normally I'd just pretend I didn't have a clue and be secretly relieved he wasn't pushing. But tonight I need to be as close to him as possible. It seems like every day I hear another story of people like us, going through hard times, who end up separating or divorcing. I need his warmth and love, the reassurance this sometimes seemingly insurmountable mountain of problems we've come upon won't tear us apart.

Hoisting my leg up almost to his waist, I dig my heel into his ass and pull him closer. For a second he resists, his body stiffening, almost bowing away. Then with a little sound, a combination moan and sigh, he relaxes and our lower bodies touch. There's the sensation of his cock, hard and unyielding, pressing against my mound, then he shifts away again.

I don't want to have to ask for sex. I want him to take over, drive all thought from my head and make me forget everything we're going through. I don't blame him if he won't though. He's too fragile right now, ego bruised by the loss of the business and shattering of our dreams. How can I fault him for not wanting to risk being shot down when we both know I've done it in the past?

"Come here." I pull him back, but softly, slowly, cupping the back of his head at the same time. Lifting my mouth to his, I whisper against his lips, "Kiss me."

He does, but gently, and I have to stop myself from making it into something feral, almost violent. A part of me wants a hard, mindless fuck, but his lips are asking for more, so I force myself to let go, sink into the sweetness of his kiss, the slow sweep and retreat of his tongue. His hand rubs and kneads my back, the motion relaxing my muscles but causing my belly to tighten with the slow warmth of building desire. The contrast is delicious, and I shiver, my nipples tingling. Pressing closer, I rub back and forth against his chest, enjoying the sensation even through two layers of clothing.

Changing the angle of his head, my husband deepens the kiss, but it's still slow—a thorough, intimate exploration of my mouth. Almost as though we're kissing for the first time, learning each other. It reminds me why just one touch of his mouth on mine can make my knees weak. One of the things he wooed and won me with was his kissing technique, and it's still as effective as ever. I can't resist moving closer, curling my fingers into his strong shoulders and enjoying the subtle movement of the muscles beneath his smooth skin.

A low hum vibrates from his mouth into mine and seems to travel through my blood to my clitoris, where it lingers, enticing me to seek further stimulation. This time when I curl my hips, sliding my pussy against the ridge of his cock, he doesn't pull away, but lets his hand drop to my ass to hold me in that position.

Still kissing, we rock against each other and let the heat enveloping us build a little at a time. This isn't a night for either haste or elaborate foreplay. Neither would truly satisfy me, and my husband knew that long before I did. That instinctive understanding of my needs is another of the myriad reasons why I love him.

When he breaks the kiss and tugs me to sit up, I go willingly, already reaching to help him slide his T-shirt off over his head. Mine is removed next, but there's still no hurry. Instead every move, each touch, is the most important moment of our lives. When he leans in to kiss and nip at my neck, it's not a prelude to anything, but an intimate, beautiful act all of its own. As my hands glide over his back, following the beloved contours, there is nothing more essential to me than the sensation of his flesh beneath my palms.

There's no sudden shift from leisurely exploration to driving desire. Instead we find ourselves sitting facing each other, now naked, my legs draped over his, our caresses no longer slow but harder, intended to take arousal to passionate, irresistible lust. Both my hands are on his cock, turning and pumping, spreading precome with each twirling sweep. His thumb circles my clitoris, pulling little moans of pleasure from me and taking me right to the edge of orgasm.

He leans in, kisses me again, and this time the contact is full of the hard-driving passion I craved before. But now the desperation I'd felt, which was born of fear, is gone. Now his demands, my equally strong responses, are natural extensions of our lovemaking, the next glorious step.

Lost once more in his kisses, my orgasm sneaks up on me, and the sound I make is equal parts pleasure and surprise. He holds me around my waist, his other hand pressing into my belly as he keeps contact with my clit, and keeps me coming and coming. By the time he stops I'm trembling uncontrollably and am practically boneless as he pulls me up onto his lap. Because of the way my legs are spread, his cock settles against my still-sensitive clit and a long, hard shudder fires through me. Pulling me close to his chest, he holds me, kisses my ear, giving me a chance to catch my breath.

Suddenly I realize the position we're in, and my heart skips a beat. This is how we made love for the first time, sitting up, face-to-face. The memory of how much I'd wanted him then fills me, sends a hot, delicious shiver down my spine. Yet, those long ago emotions are nothing in comparison to the ones flooding me now. Our shared experiences, the highs *and* lows, have given those early feelings roots and wings too, depth and strength, until I can't imagine being without him, without this overawing closeness.

Using his shoulders for leverage, I lift myself until the head of his cock finds the entrance of my pussy. His hands cup my ass, helping to guide me as I take him deep. He exhales on a long, rough breath, and his fingers tighten, trying to hold me still as he scrambles for control.

But I don't give him a chance to get a handle on the sensations. He's driven me wild, and it's time to return the favor. I rock my hips so his cock slides in and out in small increments, knowing with the angle and depth of penetration that will be enough.

"Damn, babe." He's already breathless, and his hips jerk as I rock again, a little farther out-and-back this time. "If you keep doing that, you're going to make me come too fast."

I don't bother to reply, preferring to answer with action rather than words. Besides, arousal is growing inside me again, driven by my need to pleasure him and the contact between the base of his cock and my clitoris. Trying to keep my movements slow isn't working, and

I abandon the attempt, letting go completely to rock harder, faster, allowing my body to take over and leave conscious thought behind.

The sounds he makes as his orgasm approaches, the tightening of his muscles, the way he wraps his arms around my waist, holding on as though to stop me from escaping, excite me even more. I suddenly wish the lights were on. I want to watch him come, see his face contort as his cock pulses deep inside me. I picture it in my mind just as he groans my name and thrusts up, his body stiffening and jerking with the force of his release, and the remembered image pushes me past control. I'm wild again with need, still riding him, my orgasm hovering at the periphery, teasing me.

And in that moment past and present come together with a clarity I've never experienced before, illuminating just how lucky we are, how much more important the love we share is than our circumstances. Why that revelation enters my head just then—why it's so fucking exciting—I have no way of sorting out, because I'm coming too, my arms and legs wrapped around him with convulsive strength.

Eventually we find the wherewithal to disengage, sort out the tangle of arms and legs we'd fallen into and make our way back under the quilt. Still holding him, I listen to my husband's breathing return to normal and give thanks for the marriage we've built. Life is capricious. No one can tell whether tomorrow will bring joy or sorrow. Shit can happen at any time. That's reality. The very, very best I could wish for is having a man by my side who's willing to ride it out with me, no matter what.

I have that. Recognizing the value of it, I'm suddenly more at peace than I've been for months and months.

"I'm sorry."

His whisper rouses me from my thoughts, and I tighten my grip on him. I don't want to ask, but the words come out before I can stop them. "For what?"

"For what we're going through, for getting us into this position."

I cover his mouth with my fingertips, unable to let him go on. The words resonate through me, and I shake my head.

"It's not your fault." I want to say it's mine, because deep inside that's still how I feel, but instinctively I know that won't make him feel any better. Besides, wallowing in guilt won't move us forward. I resolve to let it go, stop looking behind at what's happened and concentrate on the future. "It's not anyone's fault. We got into this together, made the decisions together. And as long as we have each other—keep loving each other—we'll make it through together."

His sigh speaks volumes. It's redolent with relief, love, contentment, and as I drift off to sleep I wrap myself in the same soothing emotions. And I'm smiling, no longer afraid of what tomorrow will bring. Whatever comes, we're stronger than it is.

We've built something that's made to last.

NOW PLAYING

CHRISTINE D'ABO

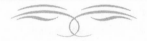

My husband and I have been together since high school, which means we've grown comfortable with each other. We complete each other's thoughts, talk in punch lines no one but us knows, and basically act as one brain. But the funny thing about growing comfortable with each other is the unfortunate side effect of forgetting that even though we know each other well, we need to take the time to reconnect and rekindle that spark that makes what we have so awesome.

I was down in the basement doing laundry when I heard the mad dash of feet upstairs and the slamming of the front door. I didn't even bother getting upset about the noise and chaos anymore. Living in a house with a teenager and a preteen meant my mantra of *stuff mom doesn't want you to do* was now automatic. I'd give them the spiel *again* when they got back in. Though where they were off to now I hadn't a clue.

I'd like to say I'm Super Mom, able to keep my cool no matter what, say exactly the right thing at the right time, all while baking cookies and working full-time. I'm not. I try, but I'm not. Normally the weekend is my time to get all the things done that I've put off through the week. Saturday was designated for running around to get errands done and buy groceries, while Sunday I reserved for laundry and housework. The routine got a bit wearing after a while, but if I didn't stick with it there were complaints of dirty underwear piling up and a distinct lack of food by Tuesday at the latest.

Frowning, I looked up at the exposed floorboards above my head. It was too quiet. I couldn't hear the kids fighting with each other, and I couldn't hear my husband stomping about either. He had his own routine on the weekends, fixing the broken bits in our house that never seemed to want to work right, helping our friends with their computer issues, or playing around on the Internet.

I'm not sure when the two of us had become so predictable, set in our ways. Maybe it came from having been together since high school, or simply because we were in survival mode, doing what had to be done just to make it to the next day. There was a time when we'd have sex on the kitchen floor, or over the back of the couch in the TV room. Long before the kids, the dogs, the mortgage and two car payments.

The quiet was unusually all consuming, prodding me into folding the shirts a tiny bit faster so I could escape the cool dark of the basement and emerge back into the sunlight. My husband's T-shirts took up half a load in the machine, the stretched cotton worn and comfortable. I had been wearing them to bed for years. He'd been pissed when I'd had to get him the next size up the last time I went shopping, claiming there was no way he'd put on that much weight. I tried telling him I didn't care even if he had. His body, while not likely to end up on the cover of *GQ*, was still capable, familiar and *mine*.

I once claimed he was built just for me. That his body stretched and changed to meet my needs, adapting as we'd gotten older. We grew and shifted together, making sure we were both happy. I don't think he believed that I still thought he was sexy despite the love handles.

Grabbing the basket of clothes, I made my way upstairs, listening for the normal sounds of our home. Even the dogs were quiet. Maybe he'd taken them out for a walk? Shifting the basket to my hip, I opened the basement door and stepped out into the kitchen. Sunlight coming in from the window washed across my face and I closed my eyes to enjoy the rare moment of peace.

The grind and pop of the garage door opening and closing had me walking farther into the room. Opening the door with a jerk, my husband practically raced inside the house, grinning like he'd just won the lottery.

"We're not suddenly rich, are we?" The basket on my hip was getting heavy, digging into my side. "Can I hire a maid? Pool boy? Can we get a pool?"

He closed the door and kicked off his shoes, apparently not caring where they landed. "I took the kids to the movies."

"You did what?" We hadn't discussed going to the movies today. Hell, I didn't even know what was playing. "Which one?"

"Don't have a clue. I bought them tickets for the first one they agreed on and gave them money for snacks." He jerked his shirt off, revealing his chest and the bulge of his biceps. I've always loved his arms. "We have an hour and forty minutes."

"For what?"

"Sex, sweetie." His grin was infectious and within a heartbeat I was smiling back at him. "I'm going to fuck you sideways."

With my husband I never knew if he was being literal or kidding. "Sex?"

"Hell yeah."

"At one thirty in the afternoon? On a Sunday?"

"You have a choice." He pushed down his shorts, leaving him in his briefs in front of the wide-open window. "I can continue to remove my shit here and I can fuck you in the living room, or we can go somewhere where we won't put on a show. I really don't care. I'm that kind of horny."

There was a time I would have laughed at the foolishness of the situation. Spontaneous sex had been something we'd indulged in early in our relationship. It hadn't been a big deal and gave us kick-ass bragging rights as a couple.

But now... God, I couldn't even remember the last time we'd fucked when it hadn't been on a schedule. We'd now gotten to a point where we had to plan our spontaneity.

I dropped the laundry basket. It could wait. "Where are the dogs?"

"Outside. They're sniffing at the bushes and peeing on the fence as we speak."

I pulled my T-shirt off and tossed it onto the basket. "That won't last long. They'll start barking at the bugs."

"Do you care?"

"Not really."

Leaving his clothing on the floor, he crossed the room and picked me up in a fireman carry. I squealed, shocked he could lift me at all, let alone throw me over his shoulder. He's not the only one who'd put on some weight over the years. He even managed to land a few slaps to my ass as he carried me up the stairs to the bedroom, though my jeans dampened a lot of the sting.

I was laughing as he tossed me to the middle of the bed, squirming myself into place. "What brought this on?"

A single push and his briefs landed on the floor, exposing his wonderfully erect cock. "I missed us."

"Us?" We talk all the time, about the kids, our jobs, the house. I yanked open the button of my jeans and lifted my hips so he could pull them off.

"I miss who we used to be. This."

And then I understood. We've both been so *busy*, it was easy to forget that before the routines, and soccer games, and daily grind, we'd been just a man and a woman who loved each other. Who craved each other's bodies and enjoyed sex. Enjoyed having fun with sex.

My bra and panties were quickly shed and I found myself finally naked. I knew I was grinning like a fool, but I couldn't help myself. "I want to be loud."

"Shit, yes."

He pushed my legs back until my knees pressed beside my breasts, opening myself up to him. I wanted to squirm away from his touch, the intensity of his gaze, but he held me still. Hot breath rolled over my pussy, causing my inner muscles to clench. He always loved going down on me, hated it when I wouldn't let him do it. I wasn't given a choice today.

His tongue was large and wet as he licked long and slow across the short hair covering my nether lips and clit. I was wet, more so than I remembered being in quite sometime, making the press of his finger into my cunt smooth as he latched on to my clit.

Every muscle in my body tensed and for a second I held back the groan. Then my brain came momentarily back to life, and I realized I didn't have to keep quiet.

I sucked in a breath and let out a long, low groan. He stopped and looked up at me, his mouth still latched to my pussy. I held his gaze and bucked my hips, encouraging him to continue. I felt his growl against my clit, vibrating. It was the last warning he gave me before losing control.

We'd been doing this for so long, you'd think it would become boring. Hell no. He knew where to push, how to crook his fingers inside me just so, pressing against the spot so I saw stars. With something as simple as a change in the routine, everything we'd been doing somehow felt new, exciting, forbidden.

My body responded faster than it had in ages. My nipples were rock hard and my skin was so sensitive to his touch. He reached up and pinched my nipple, tugging it in time to the lapping of his tongue on my clit. Every cell in my body burned, electrified. I buried my fingers in his hair, holding him in place, knowing my orgasm was going to come hard and fast. The sounds coming from him as he ate me out were obscene and cranked my arousal higher.

"Yes, fuck, right there. Don't you dare stop." There was a time when those words from me would make him do exactly that, tease and draw things out for as long as possible. But I knew he was as far gone as I was. And we still had plenty of time. We could do this again, if our bodies cooperated.

I screamed, vocalizing every bit of pleasure as he pumped his hand into my pussy while sucking hard on my clit. He moved his other hand from my breast to my hips, pressing me down into the mattress, pinning me so I couldn't shift away from the pleasure.

I had barely caught my breath, my inner muscles still twitching and grasping, when he rolled me over and pulled me onto my hands and knees. Leaning over, he nipped at my asscheek before sucking a love mark into my skin. I loved when he did that.

"I want to fuck your ass. We haven't done that in ages."

No, we hadn't. It took time and care to prep my body. Not something you can decide at quarter to midnight when we were both already sleepy. But in the bright light of the afternoon sun, I lowered my chest to the mattress and wiggled my butt in his face.

"Make it good, big boy."

Lube-covered fingers quickly found their way to my opening,

gently poking and stretching me open. He went slow, taking time to tease my clit, stoking my arousal back up so that by the time he had three fingers inside me, I was wild and panting beneath him.

"Not like this." I pulled away from him and flopped onto my back. "I want to see you."

His blue eyes were fully dilated and he was panting open-mouthed. Grabbing a pillow, he shoved it under my ass, tilting my hips to make it easier to take him. He slicked up his cock, lining himself up with me, and began to push gently forward. We'd long ago forgone the need for condoms, both of us having been fixed after the birth of our second child. It was a pleasure we'd long grown accustomed to, but never tired of—skin on skin, muscles gripping hard flesh.

I clung to him as his thrusts picked up in force and speed. With my hips tilted, my clit rubbed against his stomach.

"I love your ass. And your pussy. And tits." He leaned over me and sucked on my neck. "You fucking turn me on just by looking at me."

I sucked on his earlobe hard, knowing what it would do to him. "Harder."

His growl sounded feral, the noise rattling in his chest and vibrating through me. I knew he was close as he hooked his hands around the back of my shoulders. I lifted my legs and wrapped them around his back, forcing him even deeper. That was all it took. He threw back his head and cried out, pumping me full of his come. My muscles ached in the way that happens after great sex and I loved how he collapsed on top of me, our sweaty bodies pressed together.

I ran my fingers through his hair and pressed a kiss to his temple. "I love you."

"Love you too."

"So…the movies?"

I could feel his grin against my skin. "I figured they were old enough to go alone. Give them some independence."

"And us some time to have sex?"

"Well, I've never been one to waste an opportunity."

The sharp barking of the dogs at the back patio door bounced up the hall to our room. He sighed and started to pull out. "I'll go see what they're into."

"No. Stay." He started to protest, so I stopped him with a kiss. "They'll be fine. Let's enjoy this for a few more minutes before we have to go back to reality."

The afternoon sun warmed our bodies as a breeze caressed our skin and the dogs barked in the distance. This was our break from the norm, our chance to do something wild amidst the chaos of our lives. It was my chance to reconnect with the man I'd fallen in love with all those years ago.

I've grown to love Sunday matinees.

SEVEN

DIFFERENT FLAVORS OF LUST— EXPLORING YOUR BOUNDARIES

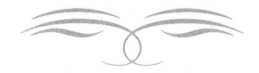

We have good sex and enough of it. We've always made a point of prioritizing our sex life and we'll let laundry pile to the ceiling before we'll skip having sex, but it's predictable, vanilla sex and sometimes I want more. We talk about our fantasies (some of them, anyway), but we never seem to get to the point of acting them out. It's like we both want to, but when we get to the bedroom we follow the script that's always worked for us.

—Natalie, married nine years

*P*oor vanilla sex, it gets such a bad rap. There's nothing wrong with traditional sex positions in familiar surroundings with no electronics, no ropes and no additional partners. There is nothing wrong with liking that kind of sex or being happy with it for the entire duration of your marriage. People use the word *vanilla* interchangeably with *predictable, routine* and *boring.* But vanilla sex is the most popular kind of sex—just like vanilla is the most popular ice cream flavor. And vanilla sex—like vanilla ice cream—is popular for a reason: it's delicious! It's what most of us have most of the time. And most of the time, we are happy with our sweet, sexy vanilla sex.

But what if you're craving something...different?

You know what I'm going to say here. The kinkiest thing any couple can do together is *communicate* their needs to each other. You don't expect your partner to know what you want for dinner every night—why would you expect him to know you want to try bondage tonight? In truth, I think most people realize they need to tell their significant others if they want to experiment outside their sexual comfort zone and that's exactly why they don't—it's outside their comfort zone. There is something scary about voicing your secret desire for a spanking, even when it's you're beloved partner you're telling. But as I mentioned in Chapter Two, if you've ever taken the plunge (with or without a little liquid courage) and shared a particularly non-comfort zone kind of fantasy, you know it's not only scary, it's kind of...well, it's *hot.* Sometimes just talking about something naughty that you've been fantasizing about is enough to get the blood pumping and the juices flowing. Sharing a sexual fantasy is the most cerebral form of foreplay and can be done whether you're with your partner or on another continent—as anyone who's ever explored the joys of phone sex, Skype sex or Google+ chat sex can tell you! (And that's a fantasy to consider exploring, too.)

One person's idea of kinky is another person's idea of an average Tuesday night (or yet another person's idea of too freaky to be considered). Don't assume you know your partner's sexual limits unless you have discussed it—and discussed it recently. People's feelings and attitudes toward sex can change dramatically over the course of a relationship and it's important to discuss what you like, what you want and what your limits are throughout your marriage. What may have made you feel uncomfortable or awkward or seemed unappealing when you were twenty-five might change five, ten or fifteen years later. I was uncomfortable about pornography in my early twenties; I'd been taught it was degrading to women and it seemed to reinforce negative body image issues I'd had since adolescence. About a decade later, after gaining the kind of confidence that comes with age and exploring the variety of porn available on the Internet, I not only made my peace with porn, I discovered that it could be even hotter when shared with my husband. We all change and grow in a variety of ways, including sexually, and that's one reason open communication is so crucial throughout a marriage. To put it bluntly: you'll never know what's possible until you ask.

Whether it's watching porn together, using ropes and blindfolds during sex, exploring male or female domination, making your own sex video, having the occasional threesome or even opening up your marriage to include other partners for one or both of you, the only way you're going to know what's okay with your spouse is to talk about it. And once you've agreed that a particular fantasy can and should become a reality, it's time to take it from discussion to action. Talking about it may be hot—but if you're both ready to try something new, you should take the plunge together.

How you proceed is going to depend on what it is you want to do. If it's something that can be accomplished with a minimum of accoutrements, you can go for it whenever you're both ready to try it. It may take a few days or weeks, as in Heidi Champa's "A Little Something Different," when a lighthearted conversation and an impulsive purchase turns a mutual fantasy of male penetration into a very scorching-hot reality. If you find that you and/or your partner are dragging your feet, telling each other "next Saturday is fantasy night" will help get you past the talking-without-doing stage. Mark it on the calendar (or set an alarm on your phone) and agree that you will commit to trying out your fantasy. Go into the experience with good humor and patience, knowing that the first time you do *anything* is bound to have a few "What do we do now?" moments. Trust me—go into it with your whole heart (and other parts) committed and you *will* get past the speed bumps. The outcome may not be what you expected—in fact, it may be so, so much more.

One plus One plus One plus… (A Note about Other Partners)

Opening up your marriage to other people requires a different kind of homework before you start. The majority of us fantasize at one time or another about people other than our spouses. If you and your spouse decide you want to make that particular fantasy reality, communication is essential. What is it you both want and agree to? A one-time threesome? Group sex? A polyamorous relationship (where one or both of you have other romantic relationships that go beyond sex and are often long-term)? There are many different possibilities beyond monogamy, and it's up to you and your partner to decide what you want. Always remember that it's the two of you at the core of any other pairings or groupings you might explore—and treat each other accordingly.

Going beyond just the two of you can be complicated and involve a variety of emotions. It's best to thoroughly explore your reasons and feelings on the subject before you take the leap. It may seem like a lot of work—and it can be—but that doesn't mean it's not worth pursuing if it's something you both feel strongly about. As Michael M. Jones writes in "Third Party," alternatives to monogamy can and do work for many couples. If you've both been thinking about it but don't know where to start, I enthusiastically recommend Tristan Taormino's book *Opening Up* and the companion website openingup.net.

Both are helpful, straightforward resources for couples interested in exploring a variety of open marriage possibilities.

Remember: whatever adventures you decide to explore together, you are the ones who make the rules for your relationship.

SENSUAL SUGGESTIONS: MIXING IT UP

Kinky means different things to different couples. Always explore your own personal boundaries with your partner in a safe, loving and playful way.

1. Skip the how-to books and go to the romance/ erotica section of the bookstore. While the stories may be pure fantasy, they will inspire lustful thoughts you can explore together.

2. Pleasing your partner, even if it's a particular kink that doesn't drive you wild, is certain to turn you on in a different way. You might discover a new kink of your own!

3. Agree to try something twice. The first time is a practice run to see how you each feel about it; the second time is the real thing. Taking the pressure off a first-time experience will keep you both relaxed and having fun.

A LITTLE SOMETHING DIFFERENT

HEIDI CHAMPA

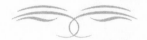

Over the years, my husband and I have shared a lot of our fantasies with each other. I always knew there was something he wanted to try that he wasn't telling me, and I tried everything to get him to open up. I realized that I had to let him come to it in his own time and in his own way. And, when he did, it was an amazing experience for both of us. When you've been together for a long time, a few little adventures can go a long way.

$\mathcal{H}$ow about something like this?"

He held up a mass of straps and cuffs that looked like dog leashes all bunched together. It was hard to tell where one piece ended and the next one began.

"What is all that?"

"Some kind of bondage kit. Looks like it's been on display for quite a while."

I shook my head and laughed as he tried to get it back on the hook. The back of the store was empty except for the two of us, the rest of the customers searching the adult DVD section for something that struck their fancy. I gazed up at the walls full of cuffs, whips and lotions, trying to find something that didn't make me cringe or giggle.

"We don't need a bondage kit. I like using your old ties. They are softer than all that nylon cording."

"True. How about this?"

It was a Kama Sutra kit consisting of a book and various potions, all in one convenient box.

"Nah. Remember what happened the last time we tried to attempt a Kama Sutra position. You nearly gave me a black eye."

"Right. Good call."

We moved in opposite directions, trying to find something for a little adventure. My eyes lit up when I got to the strap-on harnesses. I'd always secretly desired to fuck my man, but it had never come up. As a joke, I pulled one off the shelf and found a reasonably sized dildo to go with it. When I turned around, I was already laughing, fully expecting him to do the same.

"What about this, babe? Think you could handle it."

He didn't laugh. In fact, his face burned a bit pink as he cleared his throat.

"Why did you pick that?"

"I don't know. As a joke, really. Why do you ask?"

"No reason."

I walked over to where he was standing, the harness still in my hand. He barely met my eyes, instead keeping his focus on the contraption in my hands.

"Don't tell me you're interested in trying it out, Duncan?"

"Would that be so terrible, Lena?"

I tried to keep my shock under wraps, not wanting him to feel judged.

"No. It wouldn't be terrible at all. In fact, I think it's kind of hot."

I eased closer to him, letting my breasts press against his arm.

"You do?"

"Yup."

"How come you never told me that?"

"I could ask you the same thing."

"I don't know. I guess I was kind of embarrassed. I mean, I'm a guy."

"So? You've let me play with your ass before. And, it seemed to me that you really liked it."

He looked around as the last words left my mouth, a new wash of blush streaking his face.

"God, say it a little louder, I don't think the guy behind the counter heard you."

"Oh, relax. Who gives a shit what anyone here thinks? Besides, he'll know why we're buying it. The same way he knew when we bought that butt plug before."

"Very funny, Lena."

"Thanks, babe."

"This is just a bit different, don't you think?"

I pulled him into a kiss, trying to get him to relax.

"Duncan, if you're not sure, we don't have to get anything. We can just go home and have sex without any help. We can always come back and buy it another time."

He smiled and kissed me one more time.

"No. I want to buy it."

"Excellent."

For the next few weeks, there was no mention of the harness we'd bought at the sex shop. It was still in the bag, which was still on the shelf in the closet. I was beginning to think we'd spent the money for nothing. As much as I wanted to mention it to Duncan, I was waiting for him to make the first move. I didn't want to push him into anything. So, I ignored the shiny black-and-red shopping bag, although the thought of using the dildo on Duncan was never far from my mind. I was beginning to give up hope of ever getting the chance, until one night, when I came home late from work.

I could see the candlelight flickering from the open door as I walked down the hall toward our bedroom, the whole house dim and cozy. When I walked in, Duncan was already on the bed, naked with a big smile on his face. I almost laughed when he put his arms behind his head, crossing his ankles like he was getting ready for a relaxing night.

"I was beginning to think you'd never get home, Lena. I'm getting a little chilly lying here without any clothes on."

"That's why I called you to tell you I had to stay after hours."

"I didn't realize you meant a couple of hours."

"Well, I'm here now."

I crawled across the covers and planted a kiss on his grinning lips. He started to pull at my blouse, slipping the buttons through their holes quickly.

"Let's get you out of these clothes."

"Someone's impatient."

"What do you expect? I've been thinking about this for weeks now."

Even though I already knew the answer, I wanted to hear him say it.

"Thinking about what?"

He kissed me and smiled, his eyes narrowing just a bit.

"I want you to fuck me, Lena."

"Really?"

"Abso-fucking-lutely. Now, let's get you out of the rest of these clothes."

I let him slowly undress me, relishing the removal of each article of my stuffy work clothes. We twined together, making out at a leisurely pace. Duncan dropped his hand between my thighs, his fingers probing my wet slit. I gasped as one of his fingers entered me, the hardness of his cock rubbing against my thigh. I took him in hand and stroked the full length of him, the familiar gentle curve moving in and out of my fist.

"You aren't the only one who's been thinking about this for weeks, Duncan."

"I had a feeling, Lena."

I shoved him down onto his back and knelt between his splayed thighs, taking his hard cock in my mouth. His fingers ran through my hair, urging himself deeper into my throat. I couldn't resist a little tease and I slipped my finger down the crack of his ass. I pressed the pad of my finger against his pucker, doing nothing more than gently circling it. Just that little action made him gasp. I could only imagine what he would sound like when we got to the main event.

"Lena, if you don't stop, I'm going to come."

I let his cock out of my mouth with one last long lick and looked up into his glassy eyes.

"Well, we don't want that to happen just yet, do we?"

"No. Not quite yet."

I followed his gaze to the harness and the dildo sitting on his bedside table along with some lube. Something looked different about it, but I couldn't put my finger on it.

"That isn't the harness we bought, is it?"

"Nope. I took that one back."

"Why?"

"Because after doing a bit of research, I decided we needed one a little better."

I reached past him and picked it up. It looked a lot like the old one and I couldn't see what might be better about it.

"I don't get it. What's so special about this one?"

"Oh, just this."

He rummaged in the table drawer and when he turned back to me, there was a small bullet vibrator in his hand. Grabbing the harness from me, he slid the vibe inside a small, hidden pocket on the harness that would settle nicely over my clit when I wore it.

"Duncan, you didn't have to do that."

"Sure I did. I didn't want to be the only one having fun."

"Oh, don't worry, you won't be."

"Put it on, Lena. I can't wait to see you in it."

I obliged him, slipping the leather straps up my thighs and tightening the harness into place. I could feel the press of the vibe, even though it wasn't on yet. Duncan stared up at me as I attached the dildo into place. I had expected to see some fear in his eyes, but the only thing I saw there was desire.

"God, you look sexy, babe."

"Thanks. I can't lie. I feel pretty sexy too."

He sat up and kissed me, our tongues dancing for a bit before he pulled away. I watched him reach over to the bedside table and grab the lube. He pressed it into my hand, and then rolled over onto his stomach on the bed. Looking over his shoulder, he smiled at me.

"Okay, Lena. You're in charge now."

"What do you mean 'now'? I'm always in charge, Duncan."

"True enough."

I gave his ass a playful slap before I grabbed him by the hips and pulled back until he rose to his knees. Once again, I ran a fingertip over the pink pucker of his ass. My hands trembled a bit as I popped open the top of the lube bottle. I let the slick liquid drip down onto him, making him gasp.

"Damn, that's cold!"

"Sorry, babe."

"It's okay, I—"

His words trailed off as I started working the lube all around his hole, gently pressing with the tip of my finger until he let me inside. I kept adding more lube, until my finger slipped beyond his tight ring of muscle with relative ease. Duncan was propped up on his elbow, his other hand moving up and down his hard cock. I could feel the hard nub of his prostate sliding under my finger and each time I passed over it Duncan moaned a little louder. When he started rocking back against my finger, I added yet more lube and another finger. Seeing him in such a state of delight was making my pussy wetter than it had been in a long time. I was tempted to turn on the vibe in my harness, but I decided to wait.

"Are you ready for me to fuck you, Duncan?"

"Oh god, yeah. Fuck me, Lena."

I slid my hands over his ass, taking my sweet time enjoying the sight of him in front of me. It was such an odd place for me to be, but I loved it. I also took my time making sure everything was just right. The last thing I wanted to do was hurt him. I flicked the bullet vibe into action, settling it just right over my clit before I positioned the head of the dildo against his ass. Slowly, very slowly, I started pushing, and just as slowly he started to take the toy inside him. As I inched forward, the buzz against my clit got more intense. I saw Duncan tense up a bit, but I didn't back off right away.

"You okay, babe?"

"Oh yeah. Just give me a second."

I held still as he adjusted, waiting for him to move before I did.

Once again he was easing back against me, and I watched in wonder as he took the rest of the dildo inside him. Once again, we were frozen, until his words snapped me out of it.

"Please fuck me, Lena."

I did as he asked and started fucking him. It felt so different being the giver instead of the taker, the power of it all an unexpected side effect of his request. The whole thing was completely overwhelming: watching him, hearing how excited he was. That along with the vibe was sending me hurtling straight toward the edge. But I didn't want to go there alone. I increased my speed, going harder and faster. He looked over his shoulder at me and once again began to drive back against me, setting the tempo, just like he always did when he fucked me. With each thrust back, he pushed the vibe harder against my clit, my orgasm barreling down on me. Apparently I wasn't alone.

"I'm gonna come, Lena. Oh god. Oh fuck."

I watched the muscles of his back go taut, the hand working his cock moving at a furious clip. A sharp shove back from his hips put just the right pressure on my clit, my orgasm hitting me like a ten-ton truck. I moaned out his name as the second wave of pleasure crested over me, causing me to collapse onto him, my body suddenly spent from its exertion. I could hear his heavy breathing starting to slow down and the two of us fell into a heap on the bed.

After we cleaned up, we reconnected under the covers, kissing until we had to stop and take a breath.

"Holy hell that was hot, Lena."

"Yeah, it wasn't bad. So what other dirty deeds are rattling around that head of yours?"

"Jesus, woman. Give me a chance to recover."

"Sorry. I was just thinking out loud."

We lay in silence for a few minutes, his fingers lazily tracing circles on my hip.

"Well, now that you mention it, I did have a really sexy dream the other night."

"Oh really, do tell."

"Well, it all started with you in a nurse uniform."

EROTIC FICTION

THIRD PARTY

MICHAEL M. JONES

Katie and I met when we were young and foolish, in our junior and senior years of college, respectively. It was love at first sight, and we still gleefully recount the story of how I showed up on her doorstep after an eighteen-hour bus ride from Connecticut, meeting in person for the first time after a several-month courtship online (back before that sort of thing was commonplace). We've been together for almost seventeen years, married for the past fourteen. Our secret? Communication…and a mutual willingness to play outside the normal boundaries.

My wife has a boyfriend. A sweet-natured bear of a fellow some years her senior, he lives on the opposite side of the country and so they only see each other a few times a year, if that. I've met him several times, and we've chatted infrequently as the occasion rises; we even conspired to get her the perfect birthday gift one year. Like a pair of wolves, we circle each other at a distance, content to keep each other at a peaceful arm's length. He has his own family, his own loves out there on the West Coast, and I have Katie, and sometimes things overlap.

Right from the beginning, Katie and I knew we'd never be able to properly pull off the one-man-one-woman monogamous marriage. Oh sure, we had the ceremony, said the words, signed the paper, exchanged the rings. We've stuck together through thick and thin, squabbled and made up, and never stopped loving each other. At the end of the day, we curl up in bed, separated only by whichever cats have decided to act as chaperones for the night. We're mated for life, and god help anyone who doesn't understand that although we occasionally play outside the lines, the marriage still comes first. (She once threatened to defenestrate an ex of mine who didn't appreciate the rules....)

We both have wandering spirits. I've had the occasional girlfriend, Katie's had the occasional boyfriend; once in a very long while, we've even shared someone. Again, the secret is communication. We both have veto power over any prospective partner, and full disclosure is required. No sneaking around. It's not cheating if you've both rewritten the rules, right?

Which brings me back to Matthew, Katie's current boyfriend. Though they may be a country apart, they talk online constantly, and on the phone regularly. On this particular night, I was at my desk, writing as usual, pounding away at the next literary masterpiece. (I'm allowed to exaggerate, okay?) Katie was curled up on the couch, working on her laptop.

"Just so you know," she said, catching my attention, "Matt's going to call in a few minutes."

"Sounds good," I replied. I was only half paying attention, focused on finding just the right word choice, debating whether I'd find it by reading Cracked.com instead. And indeed, it was fine by me. All Katie was really doing was letting me know I didn't need to answer the phone. (I love answering the phone. Nothing breaks up the monotony of being a writer like terrorizing telemarketers, survey takers, and robots.) I went back to work.

A few minutes later, the phone rang. Katie answered, greeting Matt with the tone she uses for close friends and lovers. Her tone was low, husky, suggestive, and I had to force myself to tune it out. Out of general courtesy, I try not to listen in when she's on the phone with Matt; I don't need to know all the details, and it's a matter of trust. They chatted for a little while about the usual inanities of life—work, family, cats—and then Katie got up from the couch.

I glanced up at her movement, and she mimed going upstairs, still on the phone. I gave her another distracted wave, watching as she left the room. We've been together all of my adult life, and I never get tired of watching her walk. She's a curvy girl, with strong legs and a spectacular ass; there are days when she can hypnotize me with a wiggle and a shake. Once she was gone, I thought about getting back to work, but sadly, I belong to an easily distracted breed of writer. With my focus disrupted, it was time for a break. Feed the cats, grab a fresh drink, forage for snacks, hit the bathroom, that sort of thing.

As I wandered back down the hallway, a sound drifted down the stairwell, a low moan that grabbed my attention by the balls. Oh, I knew that sound intimately. I paused, head cocked, ears perked. A second later, another moan. Breathy and primal, and oh so familiar. I smiled, recognizing the sounds for what they were. I tiptoed to the bottom of the stairs, tilting my head so I could get the best use out of the stairwell's particular acoustic peculiarities.

"Oh, Matthew," Katie groaned. Her next words were indistinct, but the gasp wasn't. It was a short, sharp noise, followed by another low, long sound of pleasure. Something stirred within me, my cock twitching as my body responded to the undeniable sounds of my wife in the throes of passion. I've always had a voyeuristic streak, a mischievous, perverted side that comes out to play when the opportunity arises. I'd known when she went upstairs that something like this might happen—even subconsciously hoped for it. That's why I'd stopped working, why I'd wandered into the hallway, in the hopes that things might get…interesting.

I crept up the first few stairs, sidestepping the creaky one near the bottom. I paused halfway up the first flight, where I'd have a better listening point, where I wouldn't be seen. I closed my eyes, letting the sounds wash over me, painting a picture in my head. A gasp. A moan. A whimper. A low humming. Soft murmurs, almost impossible to make out. A suddenly loud "Oh god, yes! Fuck me!"

Katie has always been vocal. It's one of the things I love about her. She's not shy when it comes to expressing her pleasure. And now, as Matthew whispered words of seduction into her ear from thousands of miles away, she was touching herself, satisfying herself, making sure we both knew. She could have closed the bedroom door, but she didn't. She never does.

I closed the distance by a few more steps, still listening as she whimpered and moaned and instructed her lover to fuck her harder. "Yes!" she cried. "Like that! Oh, Matthew, yes!"

Her arousal sparked something within me, turning me on. I shifted uncomfortably, cock hard and straining to be free of my pants. I pictured her in my mind's eye, legs spread, back arched, one hand between her legs, the other barely holding the phone in place. I knew she'd reached for her Hitachi—her favorite toy—pressing it against her swollen clit, rubbing along her wet pussy. After so many years together, it's not hard to fall into a routine, to know what works for each of us. I could just imagine the flush streaking across her fair skin, lighting up face and shoulders with arousal and need. Her eyes would be closed, her lower lip caught between her teeth, her entire body rocking as she masturbated feverishly. Every sound she made was like a lightning bolt right to my libido, reminding me that I had needs too, and it had been a while since I'd done anything about it.

I quietly slipped out of my clothes, leaving a trail on the stairs behind me. Shoes, socks, pants, shirt, boxers, all discarded carelessly. Soon I was naked, erect cock springing free. I leaned against the banister, taking myself in one hand, stifling my own gasp as a charge ran through me. As my wife moaned with increasing speed and passion and loudness, I stroked myself, fingers running along the hard shaft with a light, almost teasing touch. My balls were tight with desire; I shivered as noises of arousal drifted down from the bedroom.

It didn't matter that another man was teasing my wife, fucking her by phone, driving her wild. Though he might have a small piece of her heart, she still came home to me every night, slept next to me, made love to me. And yet knowing that another man found her just as attractive, just as irresistible and desirable and sexy—it turned us both on for different reasons. It kept the fires burning, you might say.

Step by step, I slowly ascended the stairs, making it to the landing. Still out of sight of the bedroom, I again paused, leaning against the wall so I could resume stroking myself. Her cries were growing louder, more urgent, more careless, luring me in with their demanding, primal nature. I knew just how she'd arch and tense, every muscle involved, thighs tight around the vibrator as it thrummed against her sex, everything forgotten but that all-consuming need to explode. I knew the smell of her arousal, the sex-laced pheromones that even now threatened to draw me in. Poor Matt was getting an earful of her ecstasy over the phone—and why not, he'd undoubtedly earned it. Her cries rose to a crescendo before hitting one long, high, drawn-out note, a scream mixed with a whimper that signified the end of round one.

Oh yes. Katie was never one to let things end so simply if she could help it. I knew there could—and would—be more if things kept going along in this vein. Now, however, it was time for me to make my move. I finished climbing the stairs, stepped down the short hallway, then stopped, framed in the doorway. I had the perfect view as Katie slowly recovered from her orgasm, muscles loosening, body relaxing. She was naked, all of her lovely curves on display for me to see, her legs spread, sex glistening with arousal and come. One hand traced over her breasts lazily. It was a lovely, decadent sight; one that stole my breath.

She murmured soft, sweet nothings into the telephone. She glanced up, saw me standing there and shot me a wicked grin. Her eyes tracked along my body, lingering on my erection and the way I was stroking it. Like a cat about to eat the canary, she licked her lips playfully, before patting the bed next to her.

As she wrapped up her conversation, I crossed the room to drape myself on the bed next to her, stretching out. She reached over, taking my cock in one hand, even as she hung up the phone. I arched into the touch, the soft warmth of her hand so much more welcome than my own touch. "Have a nice chat, did you?" I teased.

She rolled over, still stroking me, and nuzzled in. "Of course. How much did you hear?"

"Oh, I'd say I heard plenty." A soft noise of pleasure escaped me as her fingers roamed the length of my shaft and balls, teasing and playing.

"Good. I tried to be extra loud so I'd get your attention."

"Trying to make me jealous?" I laughed. "It takes more than that, sweetheart."

"Oh no," she purred, nuzzling against my neck. "Phone sex with

Matthew's a lot of fun, and a nice change of pace, but it doesn't beat the real thing. Don't tell him, but the whole time, I was thinking about you."

"Liar," I murmured, twisting to kiss her.

"But you love me," she protested, her lips soft and warm against mine. The lingering musk of sex was strong in the air, sneaking into my nostrils, fanning the flames of my desire. She was pressed against me now, making me painfully aware of her lush breasts, sweat-slicked skin and general state of disarray. "I want your cock in me," she whispered, nipping at my ear. "I want you, thick and hard, and I want it now."

There was something raw and dirty in the way she demanded what she wanted up front; her directness always yielded the desired result. I captured her mouth in a quick, fierce kiss, before rolling over until I was on top. She was still hot and wet from her first orgasm; I was still rock hard from the voyeuristic foreplay. She guided me in with a hand, and I moaned against her lips while my cock slowly slid into her pussy. I broke the kiss in order to breathe, and she tipped her head back, eyes half-lidded. "Oh," she murmured, "God, you feel good. This is what I wanted, what I needed. You in me."

I assured her that I felt the same; that she drove me wild and was all I needed. I'm not sure how much of that was coherent, given my focus on filling her and taking my pleasure of her. She'd heard it a hundred, a thousand times before, and it was just as potent every time. I drove deep and hard, our bodies moving as one. Her nails raked along my back as I thrust into her, and my fingers dug into her sides. This wasn't a night for long, slow lovemaking; this was a time for something quick and forceful, playing off her earlier arousal and my own need for release. Her pussy was tight and wet, the perfect sheath for my cock, and I reveled in its feel. I kissed her breasts, teased her nipples with tongue and teeth while she gasped; guttural, demanding noises escaping her parted lips.

We moved together, harder and faster, and my name was on her lips as she reached the point of release again, my name turning into a keen of ecstasy to be silenced by another fierce kiss. She clenched tight around me, held me in place while the orgasms ripped through her. I felt her pulse around me, waves of pleasure rippling through her body, conducted along my cock and up into my core. "Come for me," my wife demanded, rocking against me. "I want you to come for me now."

I needed no more encouragement. A few more swift, hard strokes, and I followed her right over the edge, the last steps in a dance we'd been practicing for years. There's something to be said for the easy familiarity of an old lover or a beloved spouse, when you know each other so well and can hit the right triggers at the right moments. It was…satisfying.

Afterward, as we cuddled, my arms around her, her head against my chest, she asked quietly, "You really don't get jealous, right?" We have this talk every time, as she makes sure I'm okay with her having Matt in her life.

"Only a little," I said. "When I think of the way he gets to fire you up…but then again, I always end up reaping the benefits. I feel like I should be thanking him!"

"That might be awkward," she said with a laugh.

"Dear Matt, thanks for winding my wife up like a clockwork toy, so she takes it out on me," I teased. "Here's a beer."

She swatted my arm. "Don't you dare."

So instead I kissed her.

EIGHT

CELEBRATE YOUR LUST— SETTING THE SCENE FOR SPECIAL OCCASIONS

Holidays are crazy. We live in a different state from our families and now that we have kids, every holiday is this push-and-pull of where we're going to go, who we're going to see, who is going to come visit us. It's exhausting and frustrating and we end up getting pulled into the power plays and then bickering with each other. Every year we joke that Thanksgiving to New Year's is No Sex season.

—Matt, married eight years

W hen we're young and in love, every day is a holiday. Then reality intrudes and though we're still in love, holidays only happen according to the calendar. And then holidays become all about the kids or the extended family or needing to work overtime instead of snuggle by a cozy fire, reminiscing about our youthful days of carefree holiday lust.

Depressing, isn't it?

I don't know a single longtime married couple who haven't had a major holiday go awry. From everyone in the house being down with a stomach flu to missing a connecting flight and having to spend a holiday in a shabby airport hotel, to one spouse traveling to job interviews out-of-state while the other holds down the fort, there are times when sex not only isn't on the menu, it isn't even in the same stratosphere as what else you're dealing with. The problem is, we put so much pressure on ourselves to make every holiday perfect and to please other people that we forget about each other. We forget that, without all the love and lust that brought us together in the first place, there wouldn't be all these holidays to celebrate together.

However you choose to celebrate the calendar holidays, it's important to find time for each other. Having furtive sex at 6:00 A.M. before twenty in-laws arrive at noon for Thanksgiving dinner may not be practical (an extra hour of sleep would be practical), but it's the post-sex glow that carries us through the family fights over politics and religion, the complaints that the turkey is too dry and the fallout over The Incident at the Children's Table that will be laughed about in years to come, but not this year. And afterward, when sister Laura or cousin Bob comments on how happy/serene/relaxed we seem amidst the chaos and the cleanup, we smile and joke about drinking wine or taking a Xanax before everyone arrived. Why don't we tell the truth? "It was that amazing orgasm I had this morning with my spouse that got me through this day. Bye-bye, see you next year!" But no one wants to give grandma a coronary, so we pretend our inner glow is from the joy of spending time with family and we work very hard at not snorting or rolling our eyes when we say it.

But sometimes schedules don't work out and while it seems like the rest of the world is celebrating with party hats and sex at midnight, we're not even able to be alone with the one we love and lust for. That's a story I know all too well. My husband has been in the navy since we met and over the years we have missed every single holiday at least once—including several of our wedding anniversaries. We learned a long time ago to ignore the calendar and celebrate with each other whenever we could. Which meant Christmas fell on January 19 the second year we were married, because that's when his deployment ended, and on December 22 the year our first son was born, because that's when he had to return to his command overseas.

To be honest, I'm not even sure those are the actual dates—what I remember are a Christmas tree, presents, too much food for two people to eat, lots of laughter and—at least in the first instance—a lot of hot sex. And isn't that what holidays are all about? The two of you are the sun around which everything and everyone else revolves—or should revolve—so if relatives, children and time won't allow you to celebrate together properly, create your own holidays that are all about you and your spouse. And sex—hot, steamy, party-hat-wearing sex!

It's okay to forget the calendar, forget the traditional holidays—especially if you know there won't be time to breathe much less have any alone time—and use your imagination. Anniversaries are important—wedding anniversaries should be celebrated with as much joy and sex as you shared on your actual wedding day. But if your wedding anniversary has become a family celebration, or worse, just another workday, consider other anniversaries to celebrate: the day you met, the first time you said, "I love you," the first time you had sex, the day you committed to each other or got engaged. These are important occasions to celebrate and if you can't remember the exact dates (or some of them overlap), it's okay! You can create your own special day or days to celebrate.

A holiday can be whatever makes you feel like celebrating. Create your own calendar for just the two of you—and spend the last week of the year marking your own sexy holidays. Coordinate a sick day. Call it a mental health day and prescribe an orgasm (or two) for each other. Finally paid off your car? Celebrate the occasion in the backseat after the kids go to bed. Landed a job or got a promotion? Crack open a bottle of champagne and throw a party for two. Your youngest is potty trained at long last and you're done with diapers? Toss out the Diaper Genie and have sex on the bathroom counter. Closed on your first (or last) house? Have sex in every room! Whatever it takes, whenever you can manage it, celebrate this crazy, messy, busy life you've created together—celebrate any time you can.

We don't often get the chance to travel alone together, so my husband and I make a holiday of any opportunity for an overnight stay in a hotel. Sex in a hotel, whether it's a five-star resort or a bed-and-breakfast in a neighboring town, is a special occasion for two people who are often going in opposite directions for months at a stretch. It feels especially intimate to be cuddled up in a new bed, indulging in room service (or snacks brought along for the occasion). For a little while, time stands still and the outside world is shut away—and that is something to celebrate even if it isn't an official holiday.

But celebrating together—celebrating each other—doesn't require a trip anywhere. In an economy that has affected most of the couples I know, money is tight and holidays are a little simpler than they used to be. But as Kate Dominic writes in "Upcycling," sometimes the best Christmas gift isn't about how much you spend, it's about how much you give of yourself. This message is echoed in Heidi Champa's anniversary story, "The Next Best Thing." When an anniversary trip isn't possible, a trip down memory lane will make you feel richer than your bank balance could ever reflect.

Celebrate each other. Celebrate what got you to this point in your life, whether it's your first anniversary or your fiftieth. Even if it's only a Tuesday in the middle of the dog days of August—celebrate that passion that keeps you wanting each other and reaching for each other month after month and year after year. Call it Hot Sex Tuesday and go for it. Why? Because you can.

SENSUAL SUGGESTIONS: PARTY OF TWO

Your love and passion for each other are always reasons to celebrate. Never take for granted this amazing relationship you share!

1. Remember those "other" anniversaries—the first time you made out, had sex, got engaged, had engaged sex, whatever. Little gifts to mark those days that are special to only the two of you will strengthen your intimacy.

2. Once a month, alternate making breakfast in bed for each other. It doesn't matter if you start with Belgian waffles or Pop-Tarts—the main course is each other.

3. Give each other the gift of time. Whatever the day of the year, celebrate another day of being in love and lust with your partner. Take a moment to say, "I love you and I want you." Most of all, don't forget to say, "Thank you for choosing me."

UPCYCLING

KATE DOMINIC

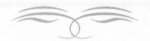

The Recession hit us hard. We (just barely) didn't lose our home, but we cut back, cut corners and counted every penny, including those in the change jar. We did it together, at first without even realizing that's what we were doing—then discovering we were very much okay with our new reality. We still had "us" and a combined bigger brain that let us figure out new, less material-oriented ways to continue enjoying not only our relationship, but the fun times we so love with our family and friends.

For over twenty years, Jeff climbed a ladder Thanksgiving weekend to festoon the house with enough lights to guide a spaceship, never mind a sleigh with reindeer, to our Southern California cul-de-sac. His dark-brown curls waved in the Santa Ana winds, his blue eyes sparkling, his muscular shoulders rippling under his T-shirt as he laughed and decorated everything from the roofline to the trees and, even after the kids were grown, the basketball hoop that still graced the garage. The Saturday after that, our party kicked off the holiday season. We feasted, danced and sang, and exchanged cookies and gifts with our large and extended circle of family, friends and neighbors. When the last reveler left, Jeff and I fucked like weasels under the Christmas tree.

Then the Recession hit. That first year, so few people RSVP'd, we almost cancelled. Instead, we hosted a quiet dinner for our immediate family and the half dozen or so shell-shocked friends who were pretty much letting our get-together be their only holiday social activity.

By the next year, after watching too many friends lose their jobs and homes, a few their marriages as well, Jeff and I weren't feeling particularly festive ourselves. He was still working, with a 10 percent pay cut and an unpaid furlough day a month. I had so few contracts I considered maintaining our vastly expanded vegetable garden to be a year-round second job. Jeff's former boss had just moved out of our den and in with his brother. The garage was full of his college roommate's furniture. My sister and her family were moving in with us after the first of the year until either she or her husband found work.

We didn't send out invitations. Still, Thanksgiving weekend, Jeff climbed up on the roof to set up a subdued light display and the inflatable Santa with sleigh and reindeer that had encircled our chimney every year since we bought the house. When he came in, his face was flushed from the wind, and he looked distracted.

"It's pretty," I smiled, handing him a cup of hot chocolate liberally laced with brandy. We'd gotten the bottle as a host gift two years ago. "But, hon, can we afford the electricity?"

"It's Christmas, dammit!" he tossed his work gloves on the table in the foyer and kicked off his sneakers. The toe was getting worn, but it would last a bit longer. "I'm sick and tired of being stressed out and depressed. Next weekend's when we've always have our party!"

He gulped cocoa, then gasped and spilled some down his sweatshirt. "Fuck, that's hot!"

It took a lot to get Jeff upset. He'd obviously reached his limit. I set my cup down beside his gloves and took his wind-chafed face in my hands. "You're hot stuff." I kissed him, running my tongue over his lower lip, tasting chocolate and brandy. His arms slid around my back and tightened, hugging me close as he parted his lips and kissed me back. He kissed me until my panties were wet.

"Sorry for snapping," he said, when we came up for air. He leaned back, resting his forehead against mine. "I'm just really disappointed."

I rubbed against him, loving the familiar swell of stiff, demanding heat jutting into his jeans.

"We can still do each other under the tree." I nipped his chin. "Multiple times. I bet we could find something to nibble besides cookies."

"Or with cookies," he laughed, licking the side of my neck. "Do we have the stuff to bake some?"

These days, I kept an inventory of every bit of food in the house. I grinned and kissed him, lots of tongue, rubbing against his erection until his eyes started to glaze. "We have everything but vanilla. Sandy next door has some. We've been swapping ingredients lately."

"Maybe we could have Dave and her over, bake cookies. Have coffee. Spice it up with booze from the cupboard. Fuck! Stop that or I'm going to come in my pants!"

"We can't have that," I murmured, dropping to my knees. I unzipped his jeans and pulled down the front of his briefs. His cock fell into my hands. I lifted it to my lips, licking slowly around the thick, warm shaft.

"Fuck." He rested his hands in my hair. The low, aroused rumble of his voice made my pussy quiver.

"What else could we do?" I took him into my mouth. He groaned and rocked his hips, shivering as I sucked his velvety soft skin over the turgid flesh beneath.

"Fuck."

Jeff's not particularly articulate when he's turned on. I clenched my thighs, my pussy creaming. I lifted off and kissed the salty tip, smiling as he trembled. "That's afterward. What else could we do—at the party?"

"Huh?" His eyes were so glazed, I doubt he heard anything but the sound of my slurping.

"Christmas lights," I said, cupping his balls. "Cookies. What else?"

"My cock in your cunt." He dragged me up and set me on the table. Cocoa splashed all over his gloves and the floor. Hot liquid pooled beneath me. I looked down and giggled.

"Fuck it," he growled, stepping between my legs. He pressed his hard-on to my crotch, kissing me until I could hardly breathe. Then he stepped back, yanking off my shoes and jeans and my sopping panties.

I lifted my legs around his waist, groaning as he slid in deep. "This is better than cookies."

He laughed and started thrusting. "This is better than Christmas!"

It was a long time before we could talk again. Eventually we staggered off to bed for a nap. The sun was low in the sky when we ended up back in the foyer, me making notes on the netbook while Jeff cleaned cocoa out of the rug. Somewhere between napping and getting up, we'd realized we were done reacting to all the crap going on around us. We were taking back control of our lives. We were having our Christmas party this year!

When Jeff stood up, I turned the netbook around and showed him the invitation.

"How does this look?"

Screw the Recession! The Christmas Party is happening!

Same place, same time as always. Some differences in how we do things.

We'll be baking cookies here, then dividing them up for everybody to take home. Bring an apron, your favorite recipes, and ingredients you already have or would be buying anyway. (Not into cooking? There will be plenty of other things to do!)

Dinner is potluck. Bring a dish to pass with 8-10 servings, again only ingredients you already have or would be buying anyway. If you want adult beverages, bring a six-pack to share or a bottle or two from your liquor cabinet. We're serious, folks! No spending money none of us have this year!

Bring your favorite holiday CDs and DVDs. Live music and performances welcome and appreciated. For those who want to go caroling, we'll be dropping off cookies instead of getting them.

We'll draw names for the gift exchange. All presents must be handmade, re-gifted, free, or a certificate for a service you provide. It's okay to swap names if what you're bringing would fit someone else better.

Holiday festive attire, however you define that—preferably something you already own. A prize will be given for best upcycling of an existing outfit.

Bottom line—no spending money! We're leaving $$ stresses at the door and having a party!

"Looks good," he said. "What the hell is 'upcycling'?"

"It's kind of like recycling, except instead of throwing something out, you restructure it into something worth a whole lot more." I hit SAVE, closed the laptop, and gave him a quick kiss. "I'll include our address, the date, yadda yadda. And I'll send e-vites, so there's no postage."

I started to step away. Jeff took the laptop from me, set it on the now-clean table and pulled me into his arms for a deep, drugging kiss.

"Thanks, babe." The smile was back in his voice. It warmed me in all the best places.

"You're welcome." I glanced around the very undecorated room and wriggled against him. "One week. Do you think we can get ready in that time?"

"Babe, I'm ready all the time."

I rolled my eyes. He swatted my butt and headed for the door. "I'll be in the garage, hauling out the rest of the decorations."

Usually we have all the prep work done long before Thanksgiving. The next seven days were a blur of coordinating, cleaning and getting ready. Except for buying mixers for the alcohol we already had or that someone else was bringing, we substituted elbow grease and do-it-yourself projects for the time-saving purchases we'd used before. At night, we fell into bed too exhausted to do more than snuggle before we were asleep.

By Saturday afternoon, the house was ready. The borrowed chairs and dishes were set out. Our second free-with-minimum-purchase Thanksgiving turkey was cooking in the next-door neighbor's oven. The au gratin potatoes were built and in the refrigerator with the cookie dough that needed to be chilled. A TransSiberian Orchestra CD was playing in the background.

My hair was up except for two deliberately curling tendrils. I'd added my grandmother's reindeer brooch to the backless scarlet dress I'd worn two years ago. I was stepping into my favorite do-me heels when Jeff came into the bedroom, cell phone to his ear.

"Joe wants to know if we need more ice—fuck!"

I pirouetted, shaking my head so the curls brushed my bare shoulders.

"Hot damn," he whispered, his gaze moving slowly over my body.

The soft wool of his suit was no match for the sudden hard-on tenting the front of his pants. "Bring whatever's in your freezer," he said into the phone. "Bring a whole fucking glacier!"

He snapped the phone shut, striding over to me—stopping just before we connected. He kissed me gently, careful of my makeup and hair. "I want to do you, right here, right now."

The doorbell rang. I slid my hand over his crotch, gently squeezing his erection. "I'm not wearing panties," I said. He groaned, took my hand and we went out to greet our guests.

It was the best party we ever had. The bakers cut out and decorated dozens of sugar cookies, made Russian teacakes, gingerbread, and toffee bars. When Jeff and a couple of his buddies started making rum balls and anatomically correct gingerbread people, they were banished to the den/man cave where they did a running, alcohol-inspired commentary for *A Christmas Story* for their vastly entertained audience.

We ate delicious hors d'oeuvres and salads, turkey and ham and all the fixings, lasagna, more side dishes than I could count, and pies and cakes. People raided their gardens and freezers and liquor cabinets. They cleared out their closets and garages to bring some truly astounding presents. Jeff ended up with a neighbor's duplicate set of metric wrenches—something he'd been wanting for a long time but never got around to buying when we had the money. I got a gift certificate from Jeff's cousin promising to build me a new raised herb bed during his holiday break from teaching. I reclaimed space in my china hutch by giving a set of German pint glasses that had been gathering dust to a colleague of Jeff's who'd taken up brewing. My sister was over the moon with our old desktop computer, now refurbished with games the neighbor's kids had outgrown. I expected that would keep everyone's adjustment to our forthcoming tight quarters considerably easier.

I brushed against Jeff whenever I could, wriggling my bottom at him. I could almost hear the wheels turning in his head, wondering if I was sashaying around the room with my pussy bare. We sang and laughed, took crazy pictures, and gave out brandy-soaked cookies as presents. It felt so good to celebrate again.

As things wound down, Jeff and I stole a few private moments on the dance floor. He slid his hand over my hip, stroking lightly through the shimmering soft fabric.

"Fuck. You're really not wearing panties." His fingers stilled. "Garter belt?"

His voice was low and deep and so very sexy. I leaned closer, smiling as his nostrils flared at the scent of my perfume. "The only things beneath my skirt are a garter belt, stockings and my bare pussy—with a drop of cherry body gel on my clit. It's getting a little itchy. Think you might be able to lick it off?"

He crushed me to him, kissing me deep and wet and hard as his erection drilled into my belly.

"We're out of here," his cousin yelled, laughing as he led the last of our guests in gathering wraps and gifts, serving platters and leftovers and cookies. A half hour later, Jeff and I stood alone in the living room, his arm over my shoulder as we sipped the last of our wine and stared at the lights twinkling on the tree.

"This was the best party ever," Jeff said, clinking his glass against mine.

"Agreed." I snuggled close, turning to rub against his still softly swollen crotch. "I think we have one more tradition to indulge in, though."

The swelling was getting hard, fast. He set our glasses on the end table. Then his hands were in my hair, cupping me to him as his tongue swept into my mouth. I tasted wine and a hint of the cinnamon cookies he'd been eating.

"Now," he growled. "Under the tree. Wearing nothing but your garter belt and stockings and your wedding ring."

My pussy juice was running down my thigh. But we took our time undressing, kissing and licking and caressing as we stripped to nothing but the attire he so loved to see framing my pussy and the gold bands on our fingers. He grabbed the afghan off the back of the couch and threw it on the rug in front of the tree. Then he eased us down, slid between my knees and lowered his face to my pussy. His tongue swept into my sopping slit.

"Cherry and pussy. Fuck, you taste good!"

I moaned and sunk my hands in his hair, the lights of the tree shimmering above me. Jeff ate me to three bucking, screaming orgasms, filling me with his fingers until I begged for his cock. With a heartfelt, "Fuck!" he rose up and buried himself balls deep in my pussy, thrusting hard and fast until I arced and wailed again. I dug my heels into his butt, my body quaking as he shuddered into me.

"Fuck. I love you," he groaned, collapsing onto me.

"I love you, too. Merry Christmas." I stroked my fingers lightly over his butt. "Let's go to bed, while we can still make it there."

He laughed and helped me to my feet. Twenty years ago, we would have slept on the floor. Tonight, our comfortable bed with its pillows and blankets was calling us. Jeff switched off the lights and led me down the hall to bed. As I snuggled into his arms, he kissed my forehead and whispered, "Merry Christmas."

I slid my hand over his crotch, squeezing his now-quiescent cock.

"Fuck," he groaned. And we were asleep.

EROTIC FICTION

THE NEXT BEST THING

HEIDI CHAMPA

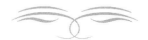

*In June of 2009, my husband got laid off from his job. It was
a shock for both of us, but it hit him particularly hard. For
the first time since he was fourteen years old, he didn't have a
job or a place to go when he got out of bed in the morning. It
started out as one of the most difficult times in our marriage,
but finding our way through made us closer and helped us
realize just how strong a bond we shared.*

"Well, it looks like we're going to have to cancel our anniversary
trip."

I turned toward him, my attention momentarily stolen from the
dirty dishes in the sink. He sat at the table, bills and papers strewn
in front of him. He took off his glasses and pinched the bridge of his
nose, a move he reserved for when he was really frustrated. I wanted to

hug him, but I was still too stunned by his words to move.

"Are you sure? We've been planning that trip for over a year."

"There's just no way we can afford it. The unemployment is barely going to cover our expenses. We just can't justify spending that much money until after I find a job. Sorry, babe."

I found myself agreeing even though I was anything but on board with his new plan. Logically, I knew he was right. Things had been tight ever since he'd gotten laid off three months prior. No more fancy dinners out for no reason, no more five-dollar cups of coffee and now, no more tenth-anniversary trip. We had spared no detail and no expense in our planning for the mini-vacation. It was supposed to be five days of bliss in the sun, sipping tropical drinks by the pool. No cares and no worries. So much for that. He moved behind as I dunked my hands back into the hot, sudsy water. It was hard not to melt into him a bit when he nuzzled my neck, but I was still reeling from the latest sacrifice that needed to be made.

"Babe, I really am sorry. But, I called the hotel and they said we could still cancel. That money is our safety net now. We can't spend it on something as frivolous as the trip. No matter how wonderful it would have been to see you in that new two-piece you bought."

"I know. I know, I know. But it still sucks."

The slow trace of his tongue over my earlobe temporarily quieted my chirping brain. When his teeth strafed over my sensitive skin, I couldn't help but gasp.

"I promise, babe. I promise you that I'll make it up to you. No matter what it takes. You'll see."

"You don't need to make anything up to me, Duncan."

"This is just a temporary setback. You'll see, Lena. Next year, we'll be sitting on that beach. I promise."

Over the next few weeks, our dream trip was the last thing on my mind. Watching Duncan come home from interview after interview dejected and miserable broke my heart every time. It was getting more difficult for him to keep his head up and while he tried to hide it, I knew it was taking its toll on him. It was hard to miss the extra scotch in his glass each night and the look of resignation on his face every time he received a phone call with more bad news.

When the day we were set to leave for our anniversary trip arrived, Duncan left the house early, planting a kiss on my forehead while I was still half-asleep. I shook the cobwebs out and focused my eyes on his face. I could tell by the set of his jaw that he was nervous. I ran my hand down his cheek feeling the smoothness of his freshly shaven face.

"Where are you going so early?"

"I have some interviews out of town. I don't want to risk being late."

I grabbed him by his tie and pulled him into a real kiss, but I could tell his heart wasn't in it. He sighed as he stood up, buttoning the jacket of his suit.

"Good luck, sweetie."

"Thanks, babe. But, at this point, I don't think luck is going to cut it."

By the time I heard the doorknob turn, signaling Duncan's arrival, I had everything set. When I met him in the foyer, his face said it all. His tie and jacket were already off.

"Hey, sweetie. How did it go?"

"How do you think?"

For a moment, I thought I'd messed up, but I decided to keep going with my plan. I pressed a cold Rolling Rock beer into his hand and took the pieces of his suit out of his grasp.

"Here, drink that. Go upstairs and change, then meet me in the living room. I have a surprise for you."

"No offense, Lena, but I'm not really in the mood for surprises tonight. And, since when do we drink Rolling Rock? We may be having a rough time, but we can still afford real beer."

"Trust me. You'll like this surprise."

I could see his resolve fading and I even detected a hint of a smile before he climbed the stairs, taking a long drink of his beer. A few minutes later, when he returned and came to the door of the living room, I heard him laugh, his body loose for the first time in weeks.

"What is all this, Lena?"

"It's your surprise. Now get over here before the pizza gets cold."

On the coffee table was the same bacon and green pepper pizza we'd enjoyed back when we were poor and living in a horrible one-bedroom apartment across town. Along with that, I'd scored us an ice-cream cake from our local grocery store, decorated with sugary roses and cheesy red writing. The Rolling Rock beer was the finishing touch. It was a staple of our college years and also the early years of our marriage when spending fifteen dollars on beer was a luxury. I had recreated our first anniversary dinner right down to the last detail, including dining at our coffee table while sitting on the floor. As he plunked down on the floor across from me, he cracked open another beer and smiled.

"I can't believe you did this, Lena. And, I really can't believe that the store still sells those cakes."

"I know it's not a trip to the beach, but I couldn't resist doing something for our anniversary. Besides, you have to admit, that night was pretty memorable."

"Very. But, if I'm being honest, it wasn't the pizza that stuck in my mind from that night."

He stood up, held out his hand to me and pulled me up to my feet. When he wrapped his arms around me, for a moment I let myself forget about all that we didn't have and focused on what was right in front of me.

"I love you, Lena. I swear we're going to get through this."

"I love you too, Duncan."

Just like we had on our first anniversary, we didn't bother to head to the bedroom. We started shedding our clothes, but I didn't get very far with my pants before he took over for me. He slid my jeans down my legs to the floor, and I stepped out of them. His hands ran back up, fingers leaving heat streaks over my flesh. My panties stood between him and my pussy, and I waited for them to be pulled down as well, but he left them. Hooking his finger in the flimsy fabric, he pulled the wet cotton aside and ran his thumb over my swollen clit. His face was close to me, his hot breath now hitting my wet folds.

"God, you are so beautiful, Lena."

His tongue dove into my pussy, my clit nestled between his warm lips. My knees nearly dropped out from underneath me, but luckily, Duncan had a firm grip on me. His hands held my hips, grinding me into his face while he licked me over and over. I felt a finger slipping between my puffy lips, coaxing my pussy open and sliding inside. One finger became two. Then three. He pulled back and just stared up at me. His fingers remained, thumb strumming over my hard clit just like his tongue had.

"Come down here. I want to watch you come."

I sank to my knees slowly; his fingers never stopped moving in my wet cunt. His mouth grazed over mine, my lips aching to be kissed. I reached out and steadied myself on his bare shoulders as my hips rocked into his hand. My body was desperate for release; the buildup from thinking about this moment all day was becoming unbearable. His eyes held mine, his fingers plunging and twisting faster and faster until my cunt clenched around them, my orgasm hitting me harder than I anticipated. As he continued to move inside me, the heel of his hand rubbing against my clit, I felt like the waves of pleasure would never stop. I rested my head on his shoulder as things started to slow down, his fingers slipping slowly out of my pussy, our lips coming together in slow kisses.

When we got to our feet, we didn't stay that way for long. I pushed him back onto the sofa and wasted no time straddling his thighs.

"Remember this, Duncan?"

"I seem to recall something like this happening that night. God, I miss our old couch. This one feels too fancy for something like this."

"Sorry, that was one thing I didn't think to recreate."

"It's okay. We'll manage with this one. Somehow."

Our laughter was quelled by our kisses, our hands roaming over each other's bodies. The head of his cock rested gently between my pussy lips, but when I tried to slide myself down, he held me so tight I couldn't move. He kissed me hard on the mouth, as I continued to struggle to get him inside me. He looked at me, his eyes dark and on fire. His lips curled into a half smile as I squirmed in his arms.

"Come on, Duncan. Quit teasing me."

"Now, where's the fun in that?"

He kissed me, running a hand through my hair as he pulled me closer, our lips still touching as I spoke again.

"Please, fuck me."

"How can I say no to that?"

He loosened his grip, and I felt myself slide down onto his cock, stretching over him until I hit bottom. Before another gasp could come out of my mouth, he crushed me with a kiss. Pushing and pulling me in his own rhythm, he moved slowly, deliberately, trying to prolong each sensation. My clit rubbed against his body, each stroke inching me closer to another climax. I closed my eyes, red and blue swirling behind my lids, my mind blank. His voice pulled me back to him.

"Look at me. Look at me, Lena."

I obeyed. I didn't have a choice. I opened my eyes, his hands holding my face, keeping my gaze on his. He pushed faster, his pace more urgent, his body tense and stiff.

"I love you, Duncan."

Just as the last word was out of my mouth, I felt my body start to tense again, my next orgasm arriving quicker than I expected. Duncan started fucking me harder, his thumbs swiping over my nipples as I started coming, gasping for air as I rode him hard and fast. It was then that I heard the telltale moan that always left his mouth right before he started to come. I looked down and saw his head against the back of the couch, his face the picture of ecstasy, his eyes pinched shut tight. We finally were still, both of us spent and exhausted. I could barely move. His chest rose and fell under me, our bodies covered in sweat. When I tried to get up, he just held me close, not letting me out of his arms.

"That was amazing, Lena."

"Yeah, it wasn't bad. It's good to see that in ten years some things haven't changed."

He held my face in his hands and gave me a sweet kiss.

"I guess the pizza's cold by now."

"Probably."

"Thankfully it's better that way. Which I believe we realized that night too."

At the mere mention of food, my stomach started to growl. Our laughter broke the spell and we pulled apart. We cleaned up and got dressed and I could tell the tension that had filled our house for so long had dissipated. We ate our cold pizza and warm beer on the living room floor and fell asleep in each other's arms for the first time in weeks, later that night.

The next morning when he walked out the door for his interview, the smile on his face said it all. It still took him a while to find a new job, but we'd found a way to make the whole process a lot more bearable.

NINE

ALWAYS TIME FOR LUST— INSPIRATION FOR YOUR OWN ADVENTURES

I wish we had a weekend to focus on each other, or even one entire night, but we don't. We have jobs that exhaust us, teenagers that are active in sports, a house we're renovating on the weekends, cell phones that are constantly ringing and beeping…there's no time for gourmet meals and bubble baths and sex marathons.

—Jackie, married seventeen years

Whether you've been married seven months, or seventeen years like Jackie, you've probably felt like that. There's no *time* for sex, much less romance, right? I understand. I really do. My marriage has been a series of military moves, long deployments, both of us working, both of us in school, book deadlines, and then, when it seemed liked life couldn't get any busier, two babies less than two years apart. I know about busy. I know about to-do lists and exhaustion and fueling up on caffeine just to get from morning to bedtime without falling asleep at a red light. I *know*.

Here is the reality: no, there's not enough time for sex. No, there's not always time for three-hour erotic fantasy reenactments. No, much as you would like to, you cannot run away to Hawaii for two weeks and leave the kids with your mother. (And if you can, most of us are kind of hating you right now.) There just isn't time every night or every week (or sometimes even every month) for all-night sex sessions. But there's always time for a quickie.

I know, it doesn't seem like much. A few stolen minutes to get it on while dinner is cooking or the shower is heating up. Nothing fancy, just bent over the counter or up against the bathroom wall, rubbing, touching, fucking. No foreplay beyond, "Do you wanna…?" and a couple of kisses to warm things up. That's what a quickie is, right? Basic, rushed, unsophisticated sex. And just when things are getting hot and heavy—well, one of you is going to be done and the other one better get there quick while there's time, before the pot boils over or the hot water runs out. Is that an accurate picture of your idea of the quickie?

Then, of course, there's the anxiety. What if it takes you longer than a meaningful fuck-me look to get turned on? What if you're so preoccupied with making sure dinner doesn't burn or the kids don't come knocking that you can't get to your happy place? What if the aliens choose that exact moment to invade the planet, while you've got your hands on your spouse's naughty bits? What if…?

Let me tell you a secret: if you wait for the perfect moment, for the night when you're both rested, healthy and not worried about work, when the dishes have been done, the house is clean, the kids are actually sleeping and not just pretending to sleep, the dog has been walked and there's no threat of alien invasion, then you will have sex twice a year, if you're lucky. And while there is definitely something to be said for quality, don't knock quantity. Here's another secret, a better one—you can have both. You can have the romantic getaway when your parents take the kids, and you leave town with only a swimsuit and a box of condoms. You can have the date night after a long, difficult workweek when all you want to do is spend time with your spouse and see a movie and have great sex after the movie, and then maybe watch another movie just because you're both still awake. You can have those intimate hours that are all about connecting and sharing and spending hours of time renewing your acquaintance with each other. And you can also have a couple of quickies a week, just to keep the emotional and sexual bonds lubricated (so to speak) and working properly.

Quickies aren't a substitute for marathon sex or date nights or romantic getaways. They're in addition to those things. Sometimes, a lot of times, they have to take the place of those things because right now, at this point in your marriage, they're all you have time for. That isn't to say you should give up on the fantasy of reenacting the Kama Sutra next weekend, or that you shouldn't buy that sex swing because you don't know when you'll have time to put it up, much less use it. By all means, indulge yourselves for as long as you can whenever you can and fantasize, fantasize, fantasize about doing more, but don't set the bar for sexual pleasure so high that you don't get to have any fun, ever. Don't look at the clock and say, "Well, we only have fifteen minutes before your parents will be here for dinner, so let's not..." Fifteen minutes is fifteen minutes! That's fifteen minutes of kissing, touching, stroking, rubbing...and connecting, not only in a physical way, but in an emotional way, too.

If making love all night is the equivalent of a gourmet dinner, then a quickie in the garage before you leave for work is the equivalent of a convenience store bag of gummy bears. Sex, like food, is all about variety. Your sex life shouldn't consist of only quickies any more than your diet should consist of only gummy bears. But life would be pretty dull without gummy bears. Or quickies.

SENSUAL SUGGESTIONS: BEAT THE CLOCK

There are times when our sex lives depend on a quickie—otherwise there wouldn't be any sex at all. Make the most of it!

1. Set a kitchen timer for ten minutes and see how far you can go. No cheating—you have to stop when the timer goes off!

2. Keep a couple's to-do list and make sure sex is on the list. It may seem silly to write "sex" under "oil change" but make your sex life as much of a priority as car maintenance, laundry and paying the bills and you'll find time for it more often.

3. The best time to have sex is first thing in the morning. Instead of hitting the snooze button, reach for your partner. It may be the best eight minutes of your day!

FOR THE SAKE OF LITERATURE

DONNA GEORGE STOREY

Sex has been an important—in fact, indispensable—part of my relationship with my husband from the beginning. In the early days, we were too busy enjoying the physical chemistry between us to talk much. As the years went by, however, I began to wish I could share deeper parts of my sexual self with my partner that could only be expressed in words. But I was shy. The stakes were too high. I realized that even two people who've done all kinds of things together in bed can have difficulty speaking openly about sexual preferences and fantasies. Then I began writing erotica and discovered an indirect, but very effective way to communicate my desires. The best surprise of all was my husband's enthusiastic response as a reader, fellow researcher and my biggest fan. It's opened a whole new level of intimacy between us. I encourage everyone to give it a try!

*I*t's Halloween night, and I'm terrified. It's not witches or zombies or sugar-crazed kids that I fear. My problem is far worse. I just gave my husband a story to read—my very first erotic story. In the final scene, the protagonist's boyfriend comes up behind her as she's washing dishes and seduces her into making love right there at the kitchen sink. The man gives orders in a smooth, assured voice—*Spread your legs, now push out your swollen lips for me, oh god, you're so tight and wet*—but in fact the semipublic sex was the woman's idea. My heroine is in the habit of leaving erotica books on her lover's nightstand with a ribbon marking the scenario she wants to explore in the flesh.

It's the dirtiest story I've ever written.

I glance over at my husband seated at our kitchen table, bathed in golden lamplight. It's a peaceful, domestic scene.

So why do I feel as if I'm about to jump out of my skin? *Is he disgusted? Embarrassed? Turned on?* I can't deny it turned me on fiercely to write it. But now I feel raw, exposed, guilty.

Desperate for a distraction, I slip into our bedroom, grab a Jane Austen novel from the bookshelf and settle in the armchair. Still I can barely concentrate. *Has he gotten to the kitchen-sink-sex scene yet? Will he think I'm a pervert?*

Finally, I hear footsteps.

"What did you think?" I blurt out, my eyes immediately darting up to his face.

His cheeks are flushed, and his lips hover on the verge of a smile. Then he glances down. I follow his gaze—and see the great, big erection tenting his jeans.

A thrill rushes through me, lifting me up off the chair and into his arms. It's as if my heart has flown right out of my chest and pulled my body along to float five feet above the floor. I laugh with pure delight.

"I can't tell you how relieved I am. Did you really like it?"

"I did indeed." He kisses me, then grins again. "But I think I should bend you over the dresser and see if I can make you come that way."

My pussy clenches like a fist. I've been so busy worrying about being judged, I didn't dare to think beyond to more enjoyable possibilities. So far the story has been all mine. Now he's offering to make it ours. My heart is pounding so hard, I'm not sure I can speak, but I manage a husky reply. "Of course. Anything for the sake of literature."

Without missing a beat, he starts instructing me, in a soft, but implacable tone, to place both of my hands on the dresser and push my ass out for him.

Trembling, I comply. His fingers fumble at my zipper. Then, just like the man in the story, he pulls my jeans and panties down to my ankles, frees one leg and orders me to spread my legs.

"Your panties are wet. Enjoying this already, are we?" Not my exact line, but close. "Well, you're going to get a lot wetter before I'm done with you. I'm going to play with your clit until your juices are oozing down your thighs."

I whimper in surprise. This part definitely isn't in the story, although I silently vow to slip it into the next draft.

My husband's hand snakes around and finds my sweet spot. I wonder, briefly, if I can actually have an orgasm this way. We've only made love in this position a couple of times, after I'd already come. But Halloween is a night for breaking rules, exploring the pleasures of the dark. Indeed it's as if he's magically pushed himself up inside my body, all the way up to my fantasy-fevered mind.

Could anything be sexier?

Why not give myself up to the sensations, his finger dancing over my clit, the other hand massaging my nipple to a point through my bra? Soon low, soft moans leak from my lips, and my thighs are slick with sweat and juice, just as he promised.

"Tell me when you're ready to be fucked. I want you to say it out loud."

"I'm ready, please, fuck me," I stammer.

"Then I'll 'press the knob of my cock into your swollen hole'? Isn't that how you said it in the story?"

The sound of my own dirty words sends my secret muscles into delicious spasm. "Yes," I whisper, blushing.

I hear him unzip, kick his pants away. A moment later he is indeed guiding his thick cock into me. I brace myself against the dresser and groan.

"Is it true what you wrote? 'As he thrust slowly, his rigid tool rubbed an exquisitely tender spot deep inside her'?"

"Yes, oh god, yes, it's true."

"Then I'm going to keep rubbing your clit and thrusting very slowly until you explode around my cock."

His voice, those words, his and mine all jumbled up together, stoke the smoldering fire in my belly. I grip his cock and rock forward and back, at just the right angle, until I feel the burn of an orgasm gathering between my legs. It is going to happen. We're going to make it real.

"I'm com...coming...pump it...hard."

He grabs my hips and rams me like a piston. I cry out, hot waves of pleasure sizzling up my torso, exploding in my skull. I come back to my senses just in time to enjoy his release, a desperate jerking of his hips in time with a flurry of deep groans.

Afterward, snuggling comfortably in our bed, he says he hopes I'll write more stories for him to read. I agree, if he promises to help me test out the scenes so I can come up with fresh, realistic images.

He smiles, his eyes glowing like candles in the darkness.

"Anything for the sake of literature."

EROTIC FICTION

THE HOTEL

MICHAEL M. JONES

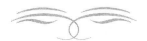

When you both work weird shifts or odd jobs, it can be rough to find time to have fun. There have been times when Katie and I only see each other as she's coming home and I'm leaving for work, or vice versa. We'll only know the other was there from a note left on the counter, or the bed already made, or a book left on the couch. Sometimes, you just have to seize the moment and take full advantage of a little free time. Take, for instance, this interlude from a period when I was working retail and it was eating my brain....

$\mathcal{I}$t was well after dark when I exited the mall and headed for my car. That was the downside of working retail and closing at the end of the night: you never got out at a decent hour. I was footsore and exhausted, and ready to go home and collapse. However, it seemed like fate had other plans in mind. There was something in my car that hadn't been there when I left it earlier in the day. There, propped pertly on the driver's seat, was a rectangular white envelope. A card. I quirked an eyebrow as I unlocked the door and picked up the envelope. There was only one other person alive who had a key to my car, and she wouldn't be caught dead near the mall without a good excuse.

The front of the envelope had my name on it, as if to make sure none of the other vast legions of people who might be getting in would think it was for them. Inside was an all-purpose "thinking of you" greeting card, one with an adorable cat and a silly saying. I flipped it open, curiously. All that was written there was, *Hotel Roanoke. Room 227.* And there was an electronic room key. My wife had struck again with another one of her spontaneously sexy, romantic moves. Either that, or I finally had a stalker. Either way, this wasn't something I dared pass up.

Twenty minutes later, I paused at the door to Room 227. The Hotel Roanoke was one of the city's oldest, finest places to stay, carrying a prestige unlike the various chain hotels. We'd lived in the city for the better part of a decade and always talked about checking it out sometime. But then again, why stay in a hotel when you have a perfectly good house nearby?

I debated whether to knock, but decided against it. I let myself in. "It's about time," came a soft, amused voice. The room was dark, lit only by a single light next to the bed, casting the rest of the plush furnishings and local artwork into shadows. There on the bed was Katie, my wife. She was sprawled luxuriously, her generous curves and soft body barely hidden by a green silk nightgown, its spaghetti straps slipping down her shoulders. It left little to the imagination, and my body leapt to the occasion, hormones kicking into high gear. My cock stirred instinctively.

Katie gave me an innocent grin, putting aside the book she'd been

reading in the meantime. (Books are our weakness, words our aphrodisiac. There are certain bookstores we're not allowed into anymore...)
"Hi!" she chirped, far too pleased with herself, and the reaction she was getting as I stared hungrily at her.

"Cats finally kick you out and take over?" I asked, trying to project a nonchalant air and failing.

She stood and walked over toward me. "I wanted to surprise you." She slipped her arms around my waist, drawing me in for a long, slow kiss; a scorcher that curled my toes and made her intentions perfectly clear. We weren't here to sleep. Oh no.

I wrapped my arms around her in return, pulling her close so I could feel the warmth of her body against mine. The silk was smooth and slippery; she wasn't wearing anything underneath. I groaned. She knew that while I love her body, I love it even more when she accentuates it with something playful and sexy. "Surprised," I acknowledged. And the time for talking was over.

She led me back toward the bed, undressing me along the way, taking every opportunity to touch and tease me. Her nails skimmed over exposed skin, followed by kisses and caresses. Every time I tried to retaliate, she lightly swatted my hands. "Not yet," she insisted. By the time we reached the oversized bed, I was naked, and she was rubbing her silk-clad body against mine, tormenting my arousal with the slick fabric and the sheer closeness of her heat. She gave me a shove; I fell backward onto the bed, sprawled awkwardly.

Her mouth was hot and wet as it took in my length, tongue swirling around my cock, teasing at the very tip as she tasted me. I threw my head back, eyes closed, and lost myself to the sensation of her mouth bobbing up and down, priming me, preparing me. Her breathing was as loud as my heartbeat. Again I reached to touch her. Again she stopped me. Instead, she released me and urged me to move backward until I was fully stretched out.

Then, meeting my gaze with a hot, burning one of her own, she lifted the hem of her silk nightgown, straddled me, and in one swift, easy motion, sank down upon me. My cock disappeared as she took it into her pussy, and her expression grew blissful. We moaned in unison as we rocked together, my wife riding my cock in a slow, steady, forceful manner. My hips arched each time, as I tried to fill her, over and over. She bent down to kiss me, while my hands slid up the inside of her nightgown to cup her breasts, thumbs brushing erect nipples. Together, we moved with increasing speed and passion until I couldn't hold back any longer. I came inside her in a powerful, profound release, and she accepted it eagerly, coaxing every last bit from me until I was spent.

Then and only then did she let me return the favor...several times.

When we were both exhausted, I managed a shaky laugh. "This was quite a surprise. How can I thank you, love?"

"Don't worry," she replied demurely. "I put it on your credit card."

EROTIC FICTION

THE KEY TO MY HEART

KRISTINA WRIGHT

It's probably no surprise that an erotica writer has an active imagination. But my indulgent, patient, sexy husband has an imagination to rival mine any day of the week. I've joked that we've tried it all at least once—and if we liked it, we tried it again.

*I*t was a crazy idea. Definitely embarrassing, potentially dangerous. Did I mention crazy? Ah, but it was too late. Once I committed—and by committed, I mean clicked the handcuff into place and tossed the key across the room—it was too late for hindsight. I had my ticket to ride, now all I could do was hold on and enjoy it. Except, my ride wasn't going anywhere.

I was handcuffed to a filing cabinet. The filing cabinet was one of those tall, industrial-metal gray types—ugly, but efficient. I, on the other hand…well, I was tall, inappropriately dressed for work and definitely *inefficient* in my current position.

The filing cabinet was in an office, the office was in a building, the building was filled with people going about their business and doing their work. Except for me—nearly naked and cuffed to the filing cabinet—and my husband, who was somewhere else. A meeting, I presumed, based on our shared Google calendar. A meeting that had ended forty-five minutes ago, about five minutes after I'd slipped into his office and out of my clothes.

I looked at the clock. Again. Where the hell was he? And why the hell had I thrown the key across the room? I didn't have an answer to the first question, but the second question was simple—I would've chickened out ten minutes into this little adventure if I had kept the key handy. Instead, it taunted me from near the door, glinting in a sunbeam from the slanted window blinds. I wasn't really in a dangerous situation. It was still early in the day and my cell phone was on top of the filing cabinet, so I wasn't "trapped" exactly, but I very much wanted that door to open and the object of my lustful plan to come walking in.

It took another couple of minutes, but the door did open and—after a moment of stark terror in which I envisioned someone else finding me—he came in. I smiled and struck a pose and…he ignored me. Rather, he didn't see me at first, with the sun in his eyes and the fact that he wasn't expecting me.

"Hey, sexy," I said, trying for a throaty seductive tone and achieving something close to an adolescent boy's warble. "I've been waiting for you."

He did the quick double take of a man who isn't quite believing what he's seeing. Then he took a little longer look. The lingerie wasn't new—a lacy black pushup bra and thong under a short pale pink slip trimmed in black lace—but I hadn't worn it in a while and definitely never in this setting. My hair was appropriately tousled in va-va-voom waves and I wore black pumps designed to be terribly uncomfortable or to show off my muscular calves, depending on who you asked. In any case, the look was having the effect I wanted because I could see his growing erection in his trousers.

"Happy to see me?" I asked, mostly because he hadn't said a word yet and I was getting nervous. Was this a mistake? His cock didn't seem to think so.

He didn't speak until he was standing right in front of me. Even then, he took a moment to finger the metal cuff around my wrist. A smile quirked at the corner of his mouth.

"So…you're my captive?"

I swallowed and nodded. I knew this man better than I knew myself. Why was the look in his eyes making me nervous? "Something like that."

"Where's the key?"

I nodded toward the door. "I threw it over there."

He glanced over at it, not really seeming to care. "So, you *are* captive until I release you."

"Um, uh, yeah, I guess so."

Not exactly the cool seductress I'd planned on being. But then, this bondage fantasy had long been one I wanted to try and assumed was more for my benefit than his. But he seemed to have gotten a decided *rise* out of it.

"Good," he breathed, leaning in close to brush the hair from my cheek. "Now what am I going to do with you?"

The natural response should've been, "Anything you want," but instead I kind of just squeaked when he raised the hem of my slip and ran his fingers along the edge of my thong.

"Already wet," he murmured, more to himself than me. "Good. I don't think I want to wait."

With that, he hiked my leg up to his hip. I was balanced on one very high heel, one wrist immobilized by the handcuffs, the other hand on his shoulder for balance. He nibbled his way down my neck to my collarbone, slipping his fingers under the cup of my bra and teasing a nipple. I shivered at all the sensations and my near helplessness.

"Unzip me."

I fumbled between us, trying to keep my balance and do as he commanded. *Commanded.* Nice word. It made me even wetter when he got all dominant on me.

"I won't let you fall," he whispered in my ear. Little did he know, I had fallen long ago and just kept falling.

I unzipped his pants and pulled his erection free. I thought to ask him to uncuff me, but then he hiked my leg higher as he pulled my panties to the side. One sweet, hard thrust into my wetness and I was flat up against the filing cabinet, the metal handles digging into my back and ass.

I yelped, attempting to shift my weight away from the file cabinet. Somehow, he maneuvered me a few inches so I was off the handles and then he got down to the business of fucking me properly. I felt helpless, desired and aroused all at once. Not to mention the added danger of someone deciding to walk in....

"Stop, wait," I gasped when he was midthrust. "Did you lock the door?"

"Why would I lock it? I never lock it."

"Go lock it," I said frantically, trying to gesture with my cuffed hand. "Before someone comes in."

He laughed. "Baby, I don't care—I'm fucking my beautiful wife in my office on my lunch hour after the meeting from hell. Let 'em look."

He smothered my protest with a hard kiss and a harder thrust. I was lost. This was what I had come here for, and I knew the risks.

Lust, like love, is filled with risks. But some risks are worth taking—
and this one most certainly was.

"Well, then fuck me and make me come before you get there," I
said, digging my nails into his shoulders.

"I thought I was in charge," he growled, on the verge of losing
control.

"Please," I added, as desperate as he was.

We got there, not quite at the same time but close enough. I
muffled my cries into his shoulder, knowing I was leaving lipstick on
his shirt and not giving a damn. He squeezed my ass in his hands as he
held me to him, silent and still as he finished what I had started.

He slowly lowered my leg back to the ground and let me get my
bearings. I smiled, feeling like the seductress I'd set out to be, as
he tucked his wet cock back in his pants and adjusted his clothes,
a smear of crimson across his shoulder. Then he stood there, just
looking at me.

I laughed, rattling the cuff. "Want to unlock me now before
someone walks in?"

"You're gorgeous," he said, emotion in his voice. "And you can
visit me at work any day of the week."

EROTIC FICTION

THE SNEAK

EVAN MORA

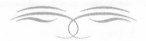

My partner and I met during a difficult time in my life: my father had recently passed away; I was going through a divorce, raising two toddlers, and trying to understand my changing sexuality. She hit me like a bolt out of the blue, and to this day I've never been more certain of anything than I am of how right we are together. That doesn't mean there weren't challenges—adjusting to being a stepparent isn't easy, and finding time to nurture a new love with a pair of rambunctious kids tumbling about requires creativity and perseverance, and perhaps, a bit of sneakiness.

There's a pitter-patter of feet in the hall outside our door. The "Quiet—shh—quiet!" of tiny voices that are anything but, and more than enough to have instantly brought me to full wakefulness. I cock an eye in Jo's direction, but she's still dead to the world.

The footsteps move on, and I track their progress: down the stairs, through the living room, into the kitchen. I hear the condiments rattle in the fridge door, then the gentle *whoomp* of the door swinging shut. A moment later, the familiar sounds of "Thomas the Tank Engine" reach my ears.

It makes me giddy—that they're down there, and we're up here. It might be as long as an hour (nearly 8:00 A.M.!) before an insurmountable obstacle brings those little feet pounding up the steps, a plaintive "Mommy?" whisper-shouted against our door.

At five and three, Ben and Lily have just learned about *the sneak*: a time-honored Saturday morning tradition involving cartoons, premade PB&J sandwiches (crusts off), milk in unspillable cups, and no parents. When I was a kid, my siblings and I loved Saturday mornings—the only day our parents slept in. Of course, they probably weren't sleeping. Clever parents.

I roll onto my side and trail a finger down Jo's arm, ready for my very own, grown-up version of *the sneak*. You see, I can't just shake her awake and tell her I'm hungry, even though I am, I always am, especially in the morning. Jo's not a morning person despite the kids, and if I move too fast she'll wake up grumpy and stumble off in search of coffee, and that will be the end of that. No, I've got to be stealthy, slide the covers down slowly, smooth my hand across her soft belly and then up to rest between her breasts. Her heart is a steady, sleepy beat beneath my palm, but it won't be for long, not if I have anything to do with it.

A featherlight caress along the curve of her breast, a teasing finger circling her areola. I lean over, brush my cheek against her softness, whisper my lips over her nipple, which hardens even in sleep. I part my lips, warm breath on her skin, and taste her with my tongue. She makes a small sound, so I do it again, swirl my tongue around the tight bud. I draw her gently between my lips, suckling her in the heat of my mouth. She moans this time, a little less asleep, but still not entirely awake.

I lean in a little closer, trade one breast for the other, lavishing it with equal attention. My hand meanwhile, is on the move, inching unobtrusively lower. Across her hip, to the juncture between her thighs where I pause, holding her intimately. She moves restlessly, pressing up against me slightly, her legs shifting to grant me better access.

I move again at her unspoken invitation, stroking the petal soft-ness of her folds, parting her gently and then dipping deeper, groaning when her arousal moistens my fingers. My clit is pulsing insistently between my thighs, my own arousal rising precipitously. I love waking her like this—with my hands and my mouth—chasing the sleep from her eyes with need. Hers. Mine. Ours together.

I find her clit and feel her breath hitch before she moans and tumbles into wakefulness. I release her breast with a reluctant kiss and smile into her warm amber eyes.

"Good morning," I whisper, circling her clit, loving the way she stretches and pushes her hips up into my hand.

"Mmmph…" she mumbles, not quite ready for speech, her hand reaching out to stroke my cheek. She licks her lips, her eyes on mine, and I press my mouth to hers. Her lips part with a gentle sigh, and I deepen the kiss, a slow tangle of tongues, still teasing her clit with my finger. What starts slow and sensual though, quickly becomes more, an urgency born of hunger and time.

"The kids?" she says against my lips as I slide my leg between hers and brace my weight on my elbow, our bodies flush from chest to thigh.

"Downstairs." I say, fingers stroking her entrance and then sliding in deep, curling up to massage her G-spot, making her arch against me. The crush of her breasts against mine makes me groan, makes my hips rock forward against her thigh, my clit hard and tight against her skin.

"You feel so good…" she breathes into my mouth, her arms sliding around me, pulling me closer still. We move together, falling into the rhythm that is ours alone, the one that's been honed through years of practice and makes us fall apart so perfectly.

"Alex!" she cries, shuddering beneath me, and I kiss her into silence as I follow. Our tremors subside and our hearts slow, and somewhere downstairs, a train whistle blows.

"That wasn't particularly stealthy, you know…" I murmur, kissing her on the nose.

"Do you think they heard?"

"I don't know."

But there it is: the sound of little feet pounding up the steps. I rest my forehead against hers with a sigh.

"Mommy?" Lily's voice is muffled, her lips no doubt millimeters from the door.

"Are you awake?" Ben's knocking loudly now, just in case we weren't.

"Is it your turn or mine?" Jo says sleepily, trying and failing to stifle a yawn.

"I'll go," I say, kissing her one last time; I'm the morning person after all. "You stay here. We'll make you breakfast and bring you some coffee." I ease out of her arms and off the bed, throwing on a T-shirt and some sweats.

"Mmph…" she murmurs, already drifting as I exit quietly and greet the troops.

"Mommy, I want—"

"Mommy, can you get me—"

"Shh…" I hunker down, finger pressed to my lips. "Mama Jo's still sleeping," I whisper conspiratorially, "shall we go and make her some pancakes?"

"Yeah!" They whisper-shout in unison, jumping up and down with excitement.

I take one of their small hands in each of mine, and together we descend to begin the next phase of *the sneak*: operation breakfast.

EROTIC FICTION

SOMEONE OLD, SOMETHING NEW

ANYA RICHARDS

The last kid has one foot out the door and suddenly my husband and I start dreaming about the freedom of it being just the two of us. Then the eldest child is laid off and constantly visiting and the middle child moves back in. Finding time for loving, and making the most of it, is priority one again.

One of the nice things about having adult children is no longer having to get up early but, unfortunately, my body apparently didn't get the memo. So I wake up at seven thirty on Sunday morning and, try as I might, can't to go back to sleep.

I slide out of bed, trying not to wake my husband. I don't do mornings, and I'm frankly peeved about my inability to sleep late. Stumbling into the kitchen, I turn on the kettle. While it's coming to a boil I resign myself to being awake and head for the bathroom to brush my teeth.

In the kitchen afterward, I'm surprised to hear my husband go into the bathroom. He's coming out as I head back down the hall, and we meet up at the bedroom door. He's smiling, reminding me how much I hate cheerful morning people, but that doesn't stop me going into his arms.

"Hi, beautiful."

I wrinkle my nose, aware of my disheveled hair and still-sleepy expression, and he grins. Leaning against the doorjamb he cradles me between his legs, bending his knees slightly so our pelvises align.

Someone woke up horny.

"Can I tempt you into coming back to bed?"

Around us the house is uncharacteristically quiet. Our kids, now young adults, keep crazy hours. There seems to always be at least one around, their din the backdrop to our lives. Much as I love them, their constant to-ing and fro-ing limits my ability to fulfill my own needs. It's worse than when they were small and in bed early. Even now I hesitate, thinking about having to be quiet in case one of them wakes up.

Then it strikes me—my stepdaughter was staying at her mother's the night before and, as I was going to bed, our youngest was going to a party across town at a friend's house.

I lean back in my husband's arms so as to see his face.

"Did Roger come home last night?"

"Nope." His hands fall to my ass, fingers pressing firmly and urging me closer. "He texted last night to say he was staying over."

Either could be home soon. There's no time to waste, but for some unknown reason I act coy. "Well." I stretch the word out to its most delicious degree. "Maybe if you ask nicely."

With a little growl he cups my cheeks and kisses me hard, demanding my acquiescence. I melt into him, desire already pulsing through my veins. The spontaneity of our encounter makes it that much sweeter. The knowledge there's no need to be quiet, discreet, makes it hotter.

I pull back slightly and caress his cock, closing my fingers around it through the cotton boxers and squeezing the way he loves. Straightening, he walks me backward across the room, stopping alongside the bed. He's already pulling up my nightie, and we break the kiss so he can whisk it off over my head. When I reach for his cock again, he grabs my hand.

"Uh-uh." He nudges me back, lowers me to the bed. "I have a plan."

"Oh?" I lie back, enjoying the show as he strips. "What kind?"

"This kind." Putting one knee on the bed, he reaches for my panties and pulls them off. I'm already wet, and when he parts my legs to stare intently at my pussy, I tremble.

With a quick shift he moves down, bracketing my legs with his arms. I want to open wider, entice him in, but when I try, he holds me still.

"Let me go, damn it."

He chuckles softly, his breath hot against my mound. "If I do, I can't do this."

With the tip of his tongue he finds the start of my slit and slides slowly lower. When he touches the upper rise of my clit my hips buck, as I try to deepen the contact. He doesn't allow it, but simply lifts his mouth away until I settle down. Once I'm quiet again, he slicks his way back to where he left off.

I can hardly stand it. The combination of his arms holding me immobilized and his talented tongue lapping at my clit already has me on the verge of orgasm. He's driving me crazy, but two can play that game.

"Fuck yeah." I don't often talk dirty to him, and he jolts with surprise. "Lick me, baby. Suck my pussy. It feels so good."

His gaze flicks up to my face, the heat in his eyes galvanizing me, but his tongue only makes another slow circle near the peak of my clit. Pressing my legs against his arms makes him tighten his grip, and I shudder, loving the gentle dominance.

"Please." I can't stop myself from begging. If I don't come soon, I'll go nuts. "Suck my clit, baby. Please."

His groan goes straight to my sweet spot, and the orgasm is already exploding in my belly by the time he complies with my plea.

He tries to go on licking me, but I grab his head, tug on it until he realizes I mean business. I tell him I want him inside me, now, and won't take no for an answer. The look on his face tells me it's going to be a hard, fast fuck, and I couldn't be happier. For the first time in a long time I make as much noise as I want, his reaction telling me he's loving it too. After I come down off my orgasmic high, I resolve to watch for more opportunities like this. They're just too good to pass up!

EROTIC FICTION

HOLDING FORTH

JEREMY EDWARDS

Some of the most significant sexual revelations in our relationship have occurred when we were away from home, outside the routine of daily life—such as during long car trips that situated us alone together with few distractions and nearly continuous opportunities for the most personal of conversations…or when we were enjoying the special atmosphere of being by ourselves in hotel rooms, with nothing but our intimacy front and center. On one occasion, I remember being on the interstate in New Jersey as we figured out something special we wanted to try in the bedroom at journey's end. That last stretch of I-80 felt much longer than usual that day!

*T*hough I hadn't exactly planned things this way, talking to Melanie about Alice that night in Toronto proved to be a door-opener—an opportunity to reveal my growing fascination with a little kink that, for whatever reason, I hadn't yet mentioned to my wife.

We'd both arranged to get out of work at noon so we could profit from an early start on our eighth-anniversary getaway. Now, after relishing the inaugural vacation-flavored drinks and dinner, we were back in our hotel room, naked in bed. It was foreplay time, and I'd volunteered to share a fresh fantasy.

"I saw Alice again today," I explained. "But let me start by asking you something about her…"

"Hey, I didn't know there was going to be a quiz!"

I managed to catch the pillow Mel had thrown at me. "It's only one question, and it's not even a trick one. Have you ever noticed how Alice always announces when she needs to pee—in so many words?"

"I don't think so."

"I mean, when we're all out having dinner and she gets up to go to the restroom, she doesn't say 'Excuse me,' or 'I'll be right back,' but always 'I need to pee.'"

"No, I guess I haven't ever noticed."

"Well, I have. And…I think it's sort of sexy."

Melanie appeared mildly intrigued. I continued.

"So the other night, after we'd been out with her, I found myself visualizing her when she has to pee…like, actually pulling down her pants in the bathroom." Just saying it made my heart speed up.

"Okay." Mel was waiting to hear what came next.

"And then this morning, she came into the museum to show me some proofs. I was on the phone, and while she waited she was checking out one of the new exhibits near my desk.

"Uh-huh…?"

"She was wearing boots with her jeans, which made those elegant legs of hers look that much longer…and when she stood there with her back to me for a minute, lingering over one of the photos, she was kind of bending one leg up behind her."

"I can see Alice in that pose."

"It was pretty hot. Likely she was doing it just to stretch or something…but I automatically imagined that she had to—um—"

"Pee?" said Melanie helpfully. The word, in her feminine voice, sent my arousal up another notch.

"Yeah, maybe she had to…pee, I was thinking, and this gymnastic act was her way of masturbating off of that—you know, her personal flavor of the 'I'll hold it a little longer' fidget."

I swallowed, very conscious of my aching hard-on, which now bobbed up from my lap. "Is that at all sexy to *you*, Mel?" I asked, feeling exposed.

She pursed her lips thoughtfully and shrugged. "Maybe a little."

I could tell this was fact, not understatement. Melanie wasn't going to get seriously turned on by contemplating a woman holding her pee; but at the right moment she might feel a slight buzz. *I'll take it*, I said to myself.

"So anyway…during the drive up here this afternoon, while you were napping, I started to spin this fantasy where Alice and I both have to pee, and—well—for some reason we have to share the restroom."

"Ooh."

Now she was definitely becoming more interested. She spooned herself more tightly to my flank, so that I could feel the loving pressure of her mound against my hip.

I clasped her left bottom cheek. As the fantasy gripped me anew, the tale came with less hesitation.

"I stand aside for Alice, but she insists that I go first. She's clutching herself—she really has to go—but she says that she gets off on holding it. And she further confesses that she gets off on watching a guy piss *while* she's holding it.

Melanie began stroking my cock.

"So I go first. And as I piss into the toilet, I turn my head to look at Alice. She's jiggling and dancing, and intently watching my stream. I finish up quickly and gesture that it's her turn—but she makes a detour to the sink. Clearly, it's an excuse to hold it even longer."

"Why that kinky vixen," said Mel with a throaty chuckle. I felt an extra quiver of excitement in my gut at this sign that she was joining more actively in the fantasy.

"She smiles at me in the mirror; and meanwhile her ass, which juts out toward me now, gyrates while she takes her time checking her makeup—she can't stand still. Her bottom looks unbelievable wriggling around in those jeans."

"Wow, sweetheart, you're so aroused."

I grunted in agreement. "Finally Alice takes her turn at the toilet. Her jeans and panties are rolled down to her boot tops. She's very graceful about it all. Her thighs are squeezed shut—but I can hear her tinkling, loud and clear. Fuck, Mel, she's pissing right in front of me, looking straight at me and sighing with pleasure."

"It must feel *so* good for her to let it flow," Melanie observed sensuously, fondling my shaft with increasing vigor.

"Oh yes. But even though I know that, I *ask* Alice if it feels good. I guess it's a way to…participate."

"Why not? It's your fantasy." She rubbed herself against me.

"Yeah," I said huskily. "And Alice replies, 'Ooh, baby,' with a wink and a wiggle. She keeps peeing for a long time, and I—"

My wife sat up abruptly. "Time out! Damn, Lawrence," she laughed, "you know what they say about the power of suggestion."

She hopped out of bed and tiptoed toward the spacious en suite bathroom.

And then, with my cock pointing after the round of Mel's derriere, I heard myself speak a question I'd wanted to ask for so long.

"Can I watch?"

EROTIC FICTION

AS FAR AS I CAN SEE INSIDE YOU

CHARLOTTE STEIN

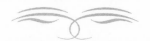

One of the best things about getting past the honeymoon stage with someone is the trust and knowledge that builds up. One minute you're fumbling and unsure, afraid to ask...the next you're doing something very naughty, in a supermarket....

He's already jiggling on the spot by the time we get to the canned goods aisle, which is a bit of a problem. Mainly because the canned goods aisle is only halfway around the supermarket. There are another five aisles to go after this, and if he's already beside himself over baked beans he's going to have major problems in the bakery.

All of those long, suggestive loaves. The smell of things rising, in the air. The sugar glistening on various glossy treats, the nipple-like tips of any number of delicacies...he's never going to make it to frozen goods. I've misjudged this badly, and trusted his word too wholly, and this is what I have to show for it.

My husband, trying to disguise his erection behind a canned ham.

He comes to the cart carrying it in the weirdest way, and of course people are looking. Which is only going to make things worse. He'd practically foamed at the mouth when I'd suggested it and fucked me into oblivion after I'd laid out the plan, so actual people staring at his lewdness must be sending him over the edge.

I'm only surprised he doesn't shove me against the shelves and take me right then and there—though I suppose this one small slip of restraint only adds to the proceedings. He must seem pretty rude to most people watching—that shape beneath his sweatpants is nearly unmistakable—but to me he's almost being coy.

He's keeping it in check, just for me, pretending to shop in this diligent, ordinary sort of way. He ticks things off the list and reaches for things that I can't get at, face hot but eyes front at all times.

It's unbearable. It's delicious. I want to lick that enormous strip of bare skin he keeps exposing whenever he does go for the top shelf—which of course makes me think he's doing it on purpose. He isn't getting things for me to be some good little shopper, as normal as the next person.

He's getting them so that I get to see the hollow at the base of his back, or the heavy slant of muscle either side of his abdomen. He knows that makes me crazy, after all. And he knows the sight of his erect cock makes me crazier—so who is this really for, when all's said and done? What is this really about?

I thought it was about him, but by the time we get to the frozen foods aisle it's increasingly about me. In truth, I thought I made him wear no underwear so that he'd be doubly mortified, doubly exposed, but now I see the truth.

I just wanted to make it easy to walk over to him, and get myself a nice, thick handful. I wanted to be able to feel him through the cloth—and I can. The ridge around the heavy head of his cock is clear, as is the curve of him, the heft of him. And if I turned just a little, stepped to one side just a little, it'd be clear to everyone else, too.

I'm shielding him, right now, as I stroke him through the material. But only just. It wouldn't take much for that old lady behind us to get an eyeful, too, and judging by the sound of his breathing he knows it.

Oh, this game has turned out even better than I thought it would. He's dancing a knife's edge of control, now, caught between public humiliation and electric excitement, and I don't know what I want more. To see him going over that edge, or to hold him there forever.

His face is beautiful, here. Flushed from temples to throat and beyond, lips parted, eyes so heavy-lidded I can barely see the blue. He has a bag of frozen peas clasped tightly in his hands, as though the cold can help him claw back some measure of restraint.

But I know it can't. I know everything about him, now, and the number one thing is this: If I push, he'll just keep going and going forever. He stretches as far as my eyes can see, a vast and near-insupportable world of sexual exploration, and for that I have to give him everything I have. When some guy catches my eye over mounds of frozen vegetables, I refuse to stop. He knows what I'm doing, and my husband knows what I am doing, and most of all, I know, too. I'm pushing my own boundaries, exploring my own sexual landscape. It looks a lot like my face suddenly pressed against his great, broad chest, so that I can hear his heart thundering as I fondle him, right out in the open. The supermarket around us narrows to nothing, and it's just me and him.

We could be alone, I think, as I stroke his gorgeous prick and hum with a stinging sort of excitement. We could be, but of course I know we're not. We're being watched, casually or not. We're surrounded on all sides and he's about to make a mess in his clingy little sweatpants—one that will be obvious, when I step away. People will point, and laugh, and stare, and maybe the store's security will come and tell us just how bad we've been.

And for a moment, I can't think of anything better. Just for a moment, just for a *second* before I let him go and his breath blows out of him all in one big blast. He's relieved, I think, but we came so close to the edge that time I know he won't be for long.

Stand on the cliff long enough, and soon you'll only be satisfied with going over. And I know this because that's how I feel, once we're back in the car park and everything is ordinary again. I want to push him over.

Then follow him down.

EROTIC FICTION

WALLS

KATE DOMINIC

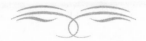

*My husband and I do live-action role-playing. The setting
for this story is accurate, and he fights in armor. However,
the story itself (at least so far) is fiction. For those reading this
who know us, if you come by our camp and scratch on the tent
door, don't be surprised to find us outside sitting around the
fire instead. What happens in the tent, stays in the tent!*

Even whispers traveled through tent walls, especially at night.
The faintest light threw shadows on the side of the pavilion that
I sure as hell didn't want anyone else seeing. This could be problematic
when Geoff and I camped with our historical reenactment group. We
liked making noise, and we liked seeing each other when we had sex.
If we timed things right, the drums and singing and general sounds
of revelry emanating from the late evening parties around the camp-

ground muffled the sounds of passion. Flames leaping from campfires distorted the shadows. On the other hand, if we went to bed too late, even deep breathing could wake the neighbors.

I'd had two cups of mead that afternoon and was feeling especially libidinous. Jeff—Geoff when he was in character—looked so damn hot in his armor. His shiny silver and leather breastplate molded his chest, showing off his broad, muscular shoulders beneath the heavy steel helm. I could damn near feel the power rippling through the air when he swung his sword.

But it was daytime. I couldn't have my way with him on the battlefield—other than in my fantasies. There were also so blasted many people awake and paying attention to everything going on around them—cooking and spinning and surreptitious cell phone conversations behind pavilions. The unspoken rules about respecting privacy included a helluva lot of simply not listening.

I decided to snare Geoff when he was done fighting. Not too soon. The clank of armor would attract way too much attention, to say nothing of my having to breathe the eye-watering aroma of a sweat-soaked gambeson that had been fermenting under armor all day. I'd catch him on his way back from the shower trucks. He'd be clean and smelling of soap and his linen tunic, maybe with a hint of beer on his breath. And he'd be amped from fighting.

I hung my dress on the back of a chair and brushed out my hair, draping myself suggestively on the bed. When Geoff pushed back the tent flap, I was wearing just my chemise and a smile.

"Hey, hot stuff." I kept my voice low and sultry, teasing my finger under the edge of my hem.

Geoff's eyes flared. He pulled the flap closed and dumped his shower gear on the rug. Then he jerked his tunic over his head. Oh yeah. His cock rose like a spear toward his belly. He lowered himself beside me, tipping onto his back.

I leaned over him, sliding my leg over his, rubbing my wet pussy against his thigh. His skin was cool from the shower, but the afternoon sun was shining on the tent. A thin sheen of sweat beaded on his body as the air around us heated and thickened.

"Come here," he growled, yanking up my chemise. He pulled me on top of him. I bit back a moan as my pussy slid over the stiff hot thrust of his cock.

Outside, an axe cracked wood. Someone was chopping kindling for the dinner fire. Someone else was clanging pots and running water.

"I want you," I whispered, grinding against him.

"You got me." He kneaded my butt with rough, scraped hands. He didn't shave when we were camping. I kissed his whiskered chin and his cheeks, swiping my tongue between his lips, catching the taste of dark ale and man.

Sometimes, I forget how truly strong Geoff is, how toned his muscles are and the stamina he has from wielding sword and shield and fighting for hours in forty pounds of steel. With no warning and no real effort, he lifted me up and turned me around. I was facing his feet, my knees on either side of his neck. He locked his hands on my hips and pulled me to his mouth. I fell forward, rubbing my face over his cock, lapping up the single salty drop running down the silky skin of his iron-hard shaft.

He rubbed his whiskers lightly over me, chafing my pussy and the insides of my thighs. His tongue slid hot and slick over my clit. I squeaked, closing my lips around his cock as he growled, "Quiet!"

I froze, wondering if I'd been too loud. But the voices outside were discussing how many turnips to put in the stew.

I groaned and took his cock in my mouth, sucking him deep as I shivered through a delicious orgasm. But Geoff didn't come. He turned me again, pulling me over him, cock to pussy, though this time with my head on his chest.

"Lift up." He patted my butt, urging me onto my knees. I reached between us, groaning as I guided him in.

More people were joining the conversation outside. Something about parsnips or carrots and how much onion to use. I rocked against him, my pussy fluttering as he twitched his cock inside me.

"I'm not going to last long." He slid one hand between us, rubbing my clit. He thrust his hips up, meeting me with each stroke. We slid against each other, slick with perspiration and pussy juice.

"Fuck!" He thrust up, arching so hard his hips lifted off the bed. I ground against him, biting back a scream as my pussy walls spasmed around him. He fell back, gasping, as I collapsed onto him.

A light scratch sounded at the door flap. "Will you be joining us for dinner tonight?"

"We're coming," we said in unison. I buried a giggle in my fist as Geoff snorted and reached for his tunic. Then he pulled on his boots and was out the tent flap while I was still braiding my hair. Somewhere in the distance, a single drummer was starting to play. I couldn't wait for his friends to join him.

LUST FOR A LIFETIME

Being married is like having somebody permanently in your corner, it feels limitless, not limited.
—Gloria Steinem, upon getting married for the first time at age sixty-six

𝒯 he stories and memoirs in this book were chosen because they reflected realistic couples finding ways to keep their sex lives fun and adventurous. I wanted to represent couples in all stages of marriage who have faced the kinds of obstacles and chaos that most couples have to deal with at some time. I wanted to give you, the curious and adventurous reader, a peek behind the closed bedroom doors of happily, lustfully married couples, and share their secrets. I also wanted to give you some inspiration and motivation—to know that you are not alone in your need for lust in your marriage, whether you've been married a couple of years or a couple of decades. You are not alone in wanting your marriage to be a partnership of hearts and minds and also libidos. You are not alone.

For years, whenever some starry-eyed romantic would ask me my best piece of marital advice, I would smile and say, "Marry someone who says yes." It's simplistic—and yet, saying yes is at the heart of every good relationship. Marry someone who says yes to you—not just to getting married or to acting out your secret sexual fantasy, but to everything your heart desires—and your life will feel limitless. Being with someone who says yes to your needs and dreams is empowering and exhilarating.

By the same token, you need to be the person who says yes to your spouse. Saying yes means putting aside your own ego, insecurities and fears and indulging his or her needs and interests. If your first instinct is to say no, you need to ask yourself why. Is it for the good of your spouse or your marriage—or is saying no about protecting yourself? If it's the latter, try to let go of whatever is holding you back and say yes. It feels *good* to say yes, to make the person you love most as happy as you can—and by saying yes, you may discover your own happiness in some new shared experience.

Here's the caveat to my advice: it only works if both people say yes to each other. Having one person who says yes to every adventure and fantasy while the other person continually shuts down any suggestion to try something new only makes for an unbalanced, resentful relationship. So say yes to each other. Every day you're married, every anniversary you celebrate, say *yes* happily and with wild abandon. Remember the person you married—and remember who you were when you got married. You are still those lusty lovers—and so much more—for your shared life together.

Enjoy the stories here and then write your own story together, whether it's in ink on the page or in whispers between the sheets. Live the story that is wholly and uniquely yours and make your lust last a lifetime. It's an ambitious and sometimes daunting goal, I know, but it's worth your time and effort, dear reader. I promise it is.

In love in Virginia,
Kristina Wright

RESOURCE GUIDE

Note: This is a collection of books and websites that the contributors to *Bedded Bliss* and I have enjoyed and found inspiring. We hope you will, too. Lusty adventures await!

BOOKS

The Adventurous Couple's Guide to Sex Toys, by Violet Blue (Berkeley: Cleis Press, 2006). (nonfiction)

Anything for You: Erotica for Kinky Couples, edited by Rachel Kramer Bussel (Berkeley: Cleis Press, 2012). (fiction anthology)

The Art of Sexual Ecstasy: The Path of Sacred Sexuality for Western Lovers, by Margo Anand (New York: Jeremy P. Tarcher/Putnam, 1990). (nonfiction)

Best Erotic Romance series, edited by Kristina Wright (Berkeley: Cleis Press, 2011). (fiction anthologies)

Confessions of a Naughty Mommy: How I Found My Lost Libido, by Heidi Raykeil (Berkeley: Seal Press, 2005). (nonfiction)

Coupling: Filthy Erotica for Couples, edited by Sommer Marsden (eXcessica Publishing, 2010). (fiction anthology)

The Erotic Edge: 22 Erotic Stories for Couples, by Lonnie Barbach (New York: Plume, 1996). (fiction anthology)

The Erotic Mind: Unlocking the Inner Sources of Sexual Passion and Fulfillment, by Jack Morin (New York: HarperCollins, 1996). (nonfiction)

The Ethical Slut: A Practical Guide to Polyamory, Open Relationships and Other Adventures (Second Edition), by Dossie Easton and

Janet W. Hardy (Berkeley: Ten Speed Press, 2009). (nonfiction)

Exhibitionism for the Shy: Show Off, Dress up and Talk Hot! (Revised Edition), by Carol Queen (San Francisco: Down There Press, 2009). (nonfiction)

Full Exposure: Opening Up to Sexual Creativity and Erotic Expression, by Susie Bright (New York: Harper Collins, 2000). (nonfiction)

Getting the Sex You Want: Shed Your Inhibitions and Reach New Heights of Passion Together, by Tammy Nelson. (Beverly, MA: Quiver, 2008). (nonfiction)

Good Porn: A Woman's Guide, by Erika Lust (Berkeley: Seal Press, 2010). (nonfiction)

How to Write a Dirty Story: Reading, Writing and Publishing Erotica, by Susie Bright (New York: Fireside, 2002). (nonfiction)

Hump: True Tales of Sex After Kids, by Kimberly Ford (New York: St. Martin's Press, 2008). (nonfiction)

Irresistible: Erotic Romance for Couples, edited by Rachel Kramer Bussel (Berkeley: Cleis Press, 2012). (fiction anthology)

The Many Joys of Sex Toys: The Ultimate How-To Handbook for Couples and Singles by Anne Semans (New York: Broadway Books, 2004). (nonfiction)

Naked at Our Age: Talking Out Loud About Senior Sex, by Joan Price (Berkeley: Seal Press, 2011). (nonfiction)

Never Have the Same Sex Twice, by Alison Tyler (Berkeley: Cleis Press, 2008). (nonfiction/fiction anthology)

Opening Up: A Guide to Creating and Sustaining Open Relationships, by Tristan Taormino (Berkeley: Cleis Press, 2008). (nonfiction)

Rock My Socks Off, by Jeremy Edwards (London: Xcite Books, 2010). (fiction, novel)

The Power of WOW: A Guide to Unleashing the Confident, Sexy You, by Lori Bryant-Woolridge (Berkeley: Cleis Press, 2011) (nonfiction)

The Ripple Effect: How Better Sex Can Lead to a Better Life, by Gail

Saltz (New York: Rodale Books, 2009). (nonfiction)

She Comes First: The Thinking Man's Guide to Pleasuring a Woman, by Ian Kerner (New York: HarperCollins, 2004). (nonfiction)

Sweet Confessions: Erotic Fantasies for Couples, edited by Violet Blue (Berkeley: Cleis Press, 2011). (fiction anthology)

Swing! Adventures in Swinging by Today's Top Erotica Writers, edited by Jolie du Pré (Logical Lust Publications, 2009). (nonfiction)

That Filthy Book, by Natalie Dae and Lily Harlem (Total-E-Bound, 2012). (fiction, novel)

The Ultimate Guide to Kink: BDSM, Role Play and the Erotic Edge, by Tristan Taormino (Berkeley: Cleis Press, 2012). (nonfiction)

The Ultimate Guide to Sexual Fantasy: How to Turn Your Fantasies into Reality, by Violet Blue (Berkeley: Cleis Press, 2004). (nonfiction)

WEBSITES

Babeland, babeland.com (sex toys and more)

Comstock Films, comstockfilms.com (website featuring adult videos of real couples)

The Erotic Woman, theeroticwoman.com (erotic fiction, photo galleries and more)

Good Vibrations, goodvibes.com (sex toys, advice and more)

Love and Sex with Dr. Laura Berman, drlauraberman.com (advice, articles and more)

Oysters and Chocolate, oystersandchocolate.com (erotic fiction and more)

ACKNOWLEDGMENTS

This book would not have been possible if not for Felice Newman at Cleis Press. I sent my proposal to her and got the kind of response writers dream of: "This is brilliant, Kristina. Truly brilliant!" I hope the final manuscript lives up to her unequivocal enthusiasm.

Thanks to all the lovely, brave, inspiring writers who contributed their stories and memoirs to the book and a special thank-you to the extraordinarily talented Donna George Storey, whose insights about cultural attitudes toward married sex sparked the seed of an idea.

Thanks to Katie Walton for her terrific research that reinforced the need for this book and to the crew at Country Club Starbucks in Chesapeake, VA for making a coffee shop feel like my home office.

Most of all, a lifelong thank-you to my husband, Jay, who has given me the roots of home, hearth and family without ever trying to clip my wings, creatively or otherwise. For twenty-three years and counting, he has been my true love and my true north and I will always fly home to him.

ABOUT THE AUTHORS

HEIDI CHAMPA (heidichampa.blogspot.com) and her husband were married in August of 1999. They've lived through seasons of plenty and times of blizzard and drought, but managed to make it through the last thirteen years of marriage with most of their sanity. Heidi is an extensively published author of erotic and romance fiction.

CHRISTOPHER COLE is a stay-at-home dad, amateur chef, part-time puppeteer and freelance writer. He met his wife of eleven years at a baseball game and though his team lost, it turned out to be the luckiest day of his life. They live in St. Louis with their three kids.

Multipublished author **CHRISTINE D'ABO** (christinedabo.com) loves exploring the human condition through a romantic lens. She has been married to her husband for sixteen happy years. Christine is published with Carina Press, Ellora's Cave, Samhain Publishing, Cleis Press and Berkley Heat.

KATE DOMINIC is a former technical writer who now writes about more interesting ways to put parts together. She is the author of over three hundred short stories, many inspired by her twenty-year marriage to the man of her dreams. They live in Southern California with their dog and several highly opinionated cats.

JEREMY EDWARDS (jeremyedwardserotica.com) is the author of the erotocomedic novels *Rock My Socks Off* and *The Pleasure Dial*. His short stories have appeared in over fifty anthologies, including recent volumes in *The Mammoth Book of Best New Erotica* series. He and his wife have been together for twenty-nine super-duper years.

MICHAEL M. JONES (michaelmjones.com) is a writer, book reviewer and editor who lives in Virginia with his wife of fourteen years. He can also be found in *Lustfully Ever After, Girl Fever, Rumpled Silk Sheets* and *She-Shifters*. He's also the editor of *Like A Cunning Plan: Erotic Trickster Tales*.

SOMMER MARSDEN's (sommermarsden.blogspot.com) erotic novels include *Boys Next Door, Restless Spirit, Learning to Drown, Big Bad* and *The Zombie Exterminator series*. Her short works can be found in well over one hundred erotic anthologies. As of February 2013, Sommer has been married seventeen years.

MARK A. MICHAELS and **PATRICIA JOHNSON** are a devoted married couple. They have been creative collaborators—teaching and writing about sexuality and Tantra together—since 1999. Michaels and Johnson are the authors of *Partners in Passion* (Cleis Press, 2014), *Great Sex Made Simple, Tantra for Erotic Empowerment*, and *The Essence of Tantric Sexuality*. Their books have garnered numerous awards: Independent Publisher Book Award, *ForeWord Reviews*, and *USA Book News* Best Books, among others. They are also the creators of the meditation CD set *Ananda Nidra: Blissful Sleep*.

EVAN MORA's stories can be found in numerous anthologies including *Gotta Have it: 69 Stories of Sudden Sex; Bound by Lust: Romantic Stories of Submission and Sensuality; Lustfully Ever After* and several volumes of *Best Lesbian Erotica* and *Best Lesbian Romance*. She lives in Toronto with her partner of six years and two children.

Multipublished author **ANYA RICHARDS** (anyarichards.com) lives with her husband of fifteen years, kids, an adorable mutt and two cats that plot world domination, one food bowl at a time. The humans support her writing while the animals see her preoccupation as a goad.

ROBIN ELIZABETH SAMPSON (erobintica.blogspot.com) is a poet, writer and blogger who's been married for more than thirty years. Her erotica, usually published under the name of Erobintica, has been included in *Coming Together: Al Fresco,* edited by Alessia Brio; *Best Erotic Romance,* edited by Kristina Wright; *Suite Encounters: Hotel Sex Stories,* edited by Rachel Kramer Bussel.

CHARLOTTE STEIN has written over fifty shorts, novellas and novels, including an entry in *Best New Erotica 10.* Her latest novella, *Make Me,* is out now from HarperCollins's new erotica imprint, Mischief. She has been with her husband for over sixteen years, and still finds herself surprised by him every day.

DONNA GEORGE STOREY (DonnaGeorgeStorey.com) and her husband have just celebrated their twenty-fifth wedding anniversary. She's published over one hundred and fifty short stories in places like *Best Women's Erotica, The Mammoth Book of Best New Erotica, Penthouse* and *Best Erotic Romance,* and is the author of *Amorous Woman,* a semi-autobiographical erotic novel.

ABOUT THE EDITOR

Described as a "phenomenal writer" by the Erotica Readers and Writers Association and a "budding force to be reckoned with" by The Romance Reader, **KRISTINA WRIGHT** (kristinawright.com) is a full-time writer and the editor of the bestselling *Fairy Tale Lust: Erotic Fantasies for Women*, as well as other Cleis Press anthologies including *Dream Lover: Paranormal Tales of Erotic Romance; Steamlust: Steampunk Erotic Romance; Lustfully Ever After: Fairy Tale Erotic Romance; Duty and Desire: Military Erotic Romance* and the *Best Erotic Romance* series. She is also the author of the erotic romance *Seduce Me Tonight*, published by HarperCollins Mischief. Kristina's short fiction has appeared in over one hundred anthologies and her articles, interviews and book reviews have appeared in numerous publications, both print and online. She received the Golden Heart Award for Romantic Suspense from Romance Writers of America for her first novel *Dangerous Curves* and she is a member of RWA as well as the special interest chapters Passionate Ink and Fantasy, Futuristic and Paranormal. She holds degrees in English and humanities and has taught composition and world mythology at the college level. Currently, she is an instructor at The Muse Writers Center (the-muse.org) in Norfolk, VA. Originally from South Florida, Kristina is living happily ever after in Virginia with Jay, her husband of twenty-three years, and their two little boys.

INDEX

INDEX